The Ultimate Guide to Pregnancy for Lesbians

•

Tips and Techniques from Conception Through Birth
How to Stay Sane and Care For Yourself

Rachel Pepper

CLEIS
PRESS

2-

Published in the United States by Cleis Press Inc., P.O. Box 14684, San Francisco, California 94114.

Printed in the United States.
Cover design: Scott Idleman / BLINK
Text design: Karen Huff
Cleis Press logo art: Juana Alicia
First Edition.
10 9 8 7 6 5 4 3 2 1

Grateful acknowledgment is made for permission to reprint the Sample Donor-Recipient Agreement on Donor Insemination from *Lesbians Choosing Motherhood: Legal Implications of Alternative Insemination and Reproductive Technologies* edited by Kate Kendell. Copyright © 1996 by the National Center for Lesbian Rights.

LIBRARY OF CONGRESS CATALOGING-IN-PUBLICATION DATA

Pepper, Rachel.
    The ultimate guide to pregnancy for lesbians : tips and
techniques from conception through birth : how to stay sane and care
for yourself / Rachel Pepper. — 1st ed.
        p. cm.
    Includes bibliographical references and index.
    ISBN 1-57344-080-9 (alk. paper)
    1. Pregnancy Miscellanea. 2. Lesbian mothers—Health and hygiene
Miscellanea. I. Title.
RG556.p47   1999
618.2'4'086643—dc21   99-22669
                                         CIP

This book is for lesbians everywhere
who dream of becoming mothers, and especially for my daughter,
Frances Ariel, who made my dream a reality.

Acknowledgments

I'd like to thank Cleis Press for jumping at the idea for this book, *Curve* magazine publisher Frances Stevens for sparking it, and my online buddies for contributing to it. Also thanks to Deborah and Dana, the wonderful midwives of Awakenings Birth Services, Anne Semans of Good Vibrations, Leland Traiman of Rainbow Flag Health Services, Kate Kendall of the National Center for Lesbian Rights, and my wonderful staff and customers at Bernal Books. I'd also like to thank Deborah Simone, Debra St. John, Tammi Goda, Cal Joy, Kristin Hofso, my parents, Joseph and Barbara Pepper, and especially Sylvia Hunt, who saw it all.

ɟ

CONTENTS

So You Wanna Be a Mamma!

Welcome to the wacky world of lesbian conception and pregnancy! I suspect, given my own experience, that you have only a vague notion at this point of what you're getting yourself into. Getting pregnant is usually harder than we ever think it's going to be before we get started. There's a lot to learn about issues of fertility and conception. There are so many decisions that have to be made about donors, sperm banks, and how we're going to define our family. Then life splits itself up into the inevitable two-week cycles of trying and waiting that could drive any sane woman mad. Even pregnancy itself, that overglorified state of female fullness, is its own roller-coaster ride of changes.

Perhaps you've always wanted to have a child, and after years of thinking about it, you're finally ready to take the plunge. Or it could be that your biological clock just started ticking yesterday, and you're already set to get busy. Maybe you're in a long-term relationship and you're both wondering how to get started on the dream you've always shared. Or maybe you're the partner of a woman who's trying to get pregnant, and luckily for her, you want to be supportive. You may even be a straight or bisexual woman fed up with mainstream pregnancy books, in which case this book may provide more of the answers that you're looking for as you try to conceive without having intercourse with a man. Whatever the case may be, the fact that you've found this book is a good first step toward realizing your goal of either getting pregnant or being there for someone who is. Believe me—either way, you'll appreciate all the help you can get!

In case you didn't realize it (but I'll bet you did!), there's a tremendous baby boom (or "gay-by boom") happening among lesbians across the United States and Canada, and in many other countries as well. A growing acceptance of gay families, greatly increased access to sperm banks and other reproductive technologies, and a noticeable surge in the urge to procreate among younger lesbians are all part of this boom. Women who live in larger urban areas may have more options for support and services, but there is no reason why, with a bit of forethought and a lot of planning, any lesbian cannot realize her dream of becoming pregnant or having a family through adoption, surrogacy, or foster parenting. While this book will concentrate mostly on the biological realities of having a child, I certainly encourage women to explore all the options open to them (and push the boundaries of options that may not initially appear so open) to bring children into their lives. We have so much love to give, and there are so many needy children already born looking for good homes, that even many women who could conceive choose to adopt or foster parent. They have my utmost respect for doing so.

Of course, lesbians have always had children. Most of these kids have traditionally been the product of heterosexual marriages. Some children of lesbians, primarily those born since the 1970s, are the result of often anonymous sperm donorship to lesbians from gay men, back in the days before AIDS. Today, with lesbian-friendly and even some woman-owned sperm banks dotting the country, most with the ability to ship anywhere in North America, the only impediments to getting pregnant, aside from fertility problems, are the cost and the time involved.

According to many sperm banks, the average length of time it takes to become pregnant with frozen sperm is about a year. Some women never do. The average cost of obtaining frozen sperm is about $300–$400 a menstrual cycle, not necessarily taking into account the cost of shipping and storage of the sperm. The narrow two-to-four-day window for conception each month puts the pressure on to make sure your timing is right, and therefore, a good basic understanding of when and how you become fertile is crucial. Whether you use fresh or frozen sperm, you should know the legal ramifications of using the type you choose, and plan accordingly with eyes wide open.

As someone who has been through this whole process, it is my hope in writing this book to provide information that's been so lacking in other pregnancy books. Although I live in San Francisco and feel that I'm both well educated and extremely plugged in to many sources of information, I have seldom felt so alienated and alone as I did while trying to get pregnant. The mainstream pregnancy books I read all seemed to assume that conception had already taken place. And the few lesbian parenting manuals on the market, while well meaning, were outdated, contained too much psychobabble, and were scarce on the nitty-gritty details of actually trying to conceive. The sperm bank I initially used seemed more concerned with profits than providing accurate information, and none of my close friends in San Francisco had ever been pregnant or could relate emotionally to what I was going through. It was a lonely time.

When I wrote an article for *Curve* magazine back in early 1998 about my experience of trying to get pregnant, the response was overwhelming. Hundreds of women from all over the world wrote me, asking about my quest and offering support and advice for what was to become my very public journey to pregnancy. This tremendous outpouring of good wishes from both women who'd been there and others just beginning their journey led me to believe that there was a very real need for a book such as the one you hold in your hands. Luckily, the good folks at Cleis Press agreed, and what was only a hunch has now become a reality.

It is with great pride that I present to you *The Ultimate Guide to Pregnancy for Lesbians*. Most of it was written during the summer I was pregnant with my daughter, Frances, and the realities of what I was going through inform every page. Also appearing throughout the text are advice and opinions from experts like Kate Kendall, director of the National Center for Lesbian Rights, who talks about some legal concerns you'll be facing, and Anne Semans of Good Vibrations, who discusses your sexual concerns during pregnancy. And you'll hear from lots of lesbian moms themselves, mostly courtesy of the gals from my lesbian parenting bulletin board on America Online. I am thankful they were there to hold my virtual hand during my own conception attempts and subsequent pregnancy.

In this book, you will first learn about your body's natural patterns of fertility, which you may never have even known existed. You'll read about sperm banks and how to pick a donor, how to inseminate at home and what happens if you do so at a clinic or a doctor's office. You'll be guided through the rough months of trying to conceive, given an honest look at the hormonal changes that may accompany your pregnancy, and be offered tips on good nutrition and self-care. All three trimesters of your pregnancy will be covered in detail, including week-by-week development of your growing baby. You'll think about options for your baby's birth, and I'll let you in on the realities of your first few weeks of motherhood. I've also included plenty of advice and empathy for the partner of the pregnant woman, because I know that as well as supporting your girlfriend, you're going through your own changes, too. There's even advice for those who just can't seem to get pregnant no matter what you try. And all this is presented with an understanding that you're a lesbian or bisexual woman—something that no other pregnancy book on this planet does!

So sit back, relax, and get ready for the ride of your life. Conception and pregnancy will be trying at times, but this book will be right there to provide encouragement, as well as answers to the inevitable barrage of questions you're bound to have. Of course, as with any health or advice book, the information here should not ever replace the advice of a licensed health care practitioner. I wish you all the best on your journey, and when the going gets tough, just remember that this book was written by someone who's been in your shoes. And if I could do it, chances are that you can too!

San Francisco
February 1999

CHAPTER 1

Thinking it Over
and Making a Plan

Deciding to have a child will most likely be the biggest personal decision you will ever make. No matter what else you do during the course of your lifetime—whether it be starting a business, moving across the country, or learning a new trade—there is nothing so profound as creating a new life. There is so much to consider when planning for a baby, but one fact remains constant no matter what your circumstances: from an abstract idea about "having a baby" will eventually grow a real live breathing creature with a personality and will of his or her own!

Your pregnancy and the birth of your baby will be a fantastic journey. At times, this journey will be filled with elation; other times it will seem maddeningly full of frustration. Before you start on this path, however, there are many questions to grapple with. Of course, these include wondering how you'll get pregnant and whether you'll use a sperm bank or donor. Still, most women begin thinking about pregnancy with a look toward the future, trying to see how a baby will fit into their world.

Among straight women, many a pregnancy is planned with the same care that lesbians bring to the process. But there are also many straight women who conceive by accident and figure out how things will work out as they go. This is usually not how we do things, because we must plan conception. So as lesbians intentionally choosing motherhood, we have the advantage of really thinking through our decision to parent and its ramifications. Although there may not ever be a "perfect" time to have a baby, some times are more perfect than others. No doubt about it, the work you will do in planning the best time and way to have your baby will go far in making you an even more wonderful mother!

Of course, there is no real way to fully prepare for the incredible and often startling changes having a baby will bring—to your relationships, to your finances, to your social life, and to you. You should be very, very sure you are aware of and willing to live with these changes before you make a baby.

The most major and stressful changes you might face when you have a baby are:

- Getting by on a whole lot less sleep.
- The possibility of ending up with a radically changed body.
- Suffering relationship turmoil if you are partnered.
- Feeling isolated, particularly if you are a single mom.
- Finding that your social and professional lives are drastically curtailed.
- Feeling worried about money.
- Not getting your own needs met.

Of course, the truly wonderful changes brought about by having a child, including tremendous love for your baby, a renewed sense of wonder in life, a greater concern for larger social issues, other people, and the planet, as well as a wonderful connection with other mothers, more than balance the scales! In addition, many of the pressure points of early motherhood ease up over the first year to a much more manageable level.

The best first step you can take when considering parenthood is to realistically assess your personal situation and contemplate how a child fits into your life. The more nitty-gritty issues of reproduction, like selecting a sperm donor, are covered in future chapters. But here are some of the biggest areas of concern for many women, and some points to ponder. I have broken them down into the areas of work, finances, your home life, your body and self-care, and your support system.

Work

Are you self employed? Work part time? Full time? If you do work full time, do you have any flexibility as to what days you work and for how long? If so, will you be able to work part time later in your pregnancy? How do you see your work life changing upon the baby's arrival? Are you planning to work full time after the baby is born? Can you afford to work part time? Will you want to work at all?

Work takes up a big chunk of our adult lives and is often a satisfying part of our self-identity. For those of us who are not independently wealthy or fully supported by our lover (or our parents, or our trust fund, or welfare), it is also how we support ourselves and our children. While many women work right through their pregnancies and rebound fairly soon after their baby's birth, others need to curtail their working hours even before the baby comes. In my own case, I was so uncomfortable by my seventh month of pregnancy that I had to cut back to working part time. As this book goes to press, Frances is six months old, and I don't know when I will ever be able to work full time again. The demands of a child are so much greater than I ever anticipated, and child care so expensive, that part-time work seems the best alternative for me right now.

Does Your Company Provide Paid or Unpaid Maternity Leave?

> *Both our employers were spectacular about our maternity leaves. I saved up my vacation time and got three months paid leave. My partner got about the same and then started back up at work part time. We are both out at our jobs, and we had no problems at all with discrimination about this.—Pam*

Most larger companies have well-defined policies about maternity leave. Make sure to find out what these are well in advance of becoming pregnant. If you can receive paid maternity leave, plan to take full advantage of what is offered, even if you don't think you'll want to. You can always go back to work early if you're ready. Recovering from childbirth can take longer than you may imagine, and it's time well spent in bonding with the baby. If you can only get unpaid leave, you will need to start saving money now to set aside for that purpose.

Are You Self-Employed?

I am self-employed and work from home. I had to start working a week after the baby was born. In a way this was easy, but in another very tiring. But I had no other choice financially.—Barb

If you are self-employed, you won't have a boss breathing down your back, but you also may not be able to take as much of a break after the baby's born. Will you close up shop for a few weeks? Or will things go on as usual, with employees running the show? If you don't already have employees, you may want to consider training someone and bringing that person on board now before you get pregnant. And is your business one to which you can take a baby? Small stores or home based-businesses work best for this. I took Frances to my book shop for the first few months of her life, but by five months she was bored with being there and part-time child care became a necessity.

Does Your Partner Get Parental Leave?

As more companies give paternal leave, they also become more open to the idea of leave for Mama's same-sex partner. Many large, progressive companies already do give at least a few paid parental leave days for nonbiological moms. To negotiate longer leave, you may have to use vacation time or take unpaid leave.

Finances

Like it or not, it is expensive to have and raise a child. Even if you plan to breast-feed and not go crazy buying lots of baby "stuff," there are lots of expenses that you won't know about till they come up. Some people have luck without much financial planning in advance, but the more usual scenario is to try to prepare a bit first. Here are some basic tips to get your finances in order:

Pay off Your Debt

If you are seriously in debt, it is wise to clear this up before you start trying to conceive. The last thing you will need during your pregnancy or baby's early life is a string of creditors knocking at the door. You may also have a harder time buying bigger-ticket items or leasing a new apartment if your credit is bad. And if your credit cards are maxed out, you may not be able to pick up the inevitable essentials (diapers, baby carrier, car seat) you will need for the baby.

Save for Childbirth

It can cost thousands of dollars to have your baby. If you are insured, find out how much of your conception and delivery costs are covered. You might also ask about coverage of infertility treatments, since these can get very costly. Now would be the time to change health plans if you need to. If you have to pay hospital costs for delivery or intend to have a home birth with a midwife, you are probably going to need about $2,000 for a basic delivery. If you have complications during labor, the costs will be even higher.

Post-Baby Savings

If you are able to, save a little something for after the baby's born. It is harder than you would expect to go back to work after the baby comes. Your body needs healing and your baby needs your company. You should plan on a maternity leave of at least a month. I needed about six weeks before I was ready to head back out into the world. How will you support yourself during this time? Maybe your partner will be paying the bills, or your parents will help. But if you are on your own, you should plan on having at least an extra month's rent, utilities, and grocery money set aside. As I will discuss later in the book, you should also plan to have some money set aside for doula care, especially if you are a single mama or your partner will be working full time after the baby arrives. A doula is a professional labor assistant who will provide guidance and support before, during, and after the baby's birth. See chapters 7 and 11 for more on doulas.

Home Life

One of the best gifts you can give your child is a happy, stable home life. It doesn't matter if you are in a coupled relationship or not. What does matter is if you are truly ready to welcome another person into your family, no matter what its size or makeup. You should first ask yourself if you are ready emotionally to care for a child. Gotten the travel bug out of your system for a while? No need to go out partying for at least a few months? Worked out some of those pesky personal issues that plague us all? Feeling in control of your life and the direction it's going? Good!

Now it's time to look at those around you:

Roommates

If you live with roommates, you should be honest with them about your plans to conceive. If they seem less than enthusiastic, or are in any way unfit to live with a young child, you might want to find a new dwelling, or ask them to.

Girlfriends

If you are in a relationship with another woman and you have doubts about the stability of your union, it may not be the best time to try to get pregnant. Don't make the same mistake some straight couples do and think having a child will "save" the relationship. If you are in a committed relationship and are planning the baby together, make sure you have similar expectations for what this will mean—now and for the next twenty years.

Living Alone

If you are unpartnered or just live alone, you can set up the kind of home that you want for yourself and baby. Just make sure you line up enough support for yourself after the baby's born.

Body and Self-Care

Women of all different body types, weights, and physical abilities can conceive, give birth, and become good mothers. But because pregnancy is often physically and emotionally draining, it pays to be in the best shape you can be before you begin to inseminate. Eating well, drinking lots of water, quitting smoking, cutting back on caffeine and alcohol, and exercising regularly are all good preparation for pregnancy. You should talk to your doctor about any prescription medicines you are taking and decide whether you might be able to go off them for the duration of your pregnancy.

Self-care is very important during both the conception process and pregnancy. The better you take care of yourself, the better your odds of enjoying your pregnancy and delivering a healthy baby.

Safer Sex

Now is the time to review your safer-sex practices. Many sexually transmitted diseases, such as HIV, chlamydia, and herpes, can be passed along to the fetus or can complicate pregnancy.

Naturally, you will have a complete gynecological checkup, including tests for HIV, hepatitis B and C, chlamydia, gonnorhea, syphilis, herpes, and so on. While you are trying to get pregnant, be extra vigilant about your sexual health.

If you and your girlfriend have sex only with each other and have tested negative for HIV and other STDs, your safer-sex requirements are much simplified. Here are a few guidelines to keep in mind:

- Remember that your girlfriend needs to keep up her gynecological care, too. "Fluid-bonding" works only if you both commit to good health practices. A pesky vaginal infection can be transmitted through oral sex.
- Keep your toys clean. Use condoms on dildos and vibrators to prevent sharing vaginal infections.
- Do not allow anal bacteria access to the vagina. After anal sex and before vaginal sex, wash your hands, rinse your mouth, discard that latex glove or condom, and clean your toys.
- Do not used oil-based lubricants (like Crisco, Vaseline, or baby oil) for vaginal penetration. Oil-based lube does not rinse out of the vagina very easily and thus provides a great breeding ground for vaginal infections. Use water-based lubes instead.

If you have more than one sex partner or if you or your partner may have been exposed to an STD, it's time to make some decisions about safer-sex practices.

Most safer-sex recommendations are geared toward sex with men. Cautions abound regarding anal and vaginal penetration with a condomless penis. But what about sex between women? What is safe? How do you assess your risk and make informed decisions? The fact is that unprotected sex between women *can* transmit STDs—particularly cunnilingus, particularly during menstruation. Educate yourself, talk with your girlfriend(s), and make informed decisions for your health.

Conditions for Concern

In some ways, I think having a high risk pregnancy had its real advantages. We saw the doctor frequently and never went long without a question being answered. In the end, I suspect that I had a healthier pregnancy than many women. — Joanne

If you think you may be a candidate for a "high-risk" pregnancy because of existing health problems, you should consult a doctor or other trusted health care professional before you begin to inseminate. Diabetes, which came up often among women I talked to in researching this book, is a good example of a condition you may need to monitor closely during pregnancy. You may also need to closely monitor your pregnancy if you have had previous abortions, miscarriage, or past problems with your reproductive tract, including endometriosis or an ectopic pregnancy, where the fertilized egg implants in a fallopian tube instead of the uterus. If you are over forty years old, your health care provider may also want to watch you carefully, since you will have a greater risk of miscarriage and of having a baby born with Down's syndrome. While some women go into pregnancy knowing they may have a more difficult time, don't forget that any pregnancy can become high risk. Conditions such as placenta previa, where the placenta blocks the cervix, or preeclampsia, where the women develops high blood pressure, can strike any woman during her pregnancy. With careful monitoring, however, most such conditions don't interfere with a woman's ability to carry her baby to term.

Friends told us that pregnancy with a condition like diabetes is like the normal experience of pregnancy times ten. We were very dependent on a competent and up-to-date medical team who supported our decision to get pregnant. We were so glad that we had each other and that our team respected our decisions.—Nicca

I have a history of diabetes and although I was very healthy at the time I got pregnant, I fully expected gestational diabetes. At eighteen weeks, that diagnosis was confirmed.—Yvonne

I think being an older mom actually was easier for me. Because I'm in my forties, I'm more educated about how the medical system works and was better able to advocate for myself. I eat well, don't drink anymore, and take really good care of myself, which is more than I can say about how I lived in my twenties and thirties. Although it took me over a year to get pregnant, I had few complications and had an easy delivery.—Joanne

If you live with a condition such as diabetes, talk to other women who have had a similar experiences and find a doctor who believes in your ability to have a normal pregnancy with as little intervention as you prefer. If you are over forty, consider joining a support group for other "older" moms and find out as much as you can about how to keep yourself as healthy as possible.

RECOMMENDED READING

Past Due:
A Story of
Disability,
Pregnancy, and
Birth
by Anne Finger.

Disability

There are many types of physical conditions labeled by larger society as "disabilities." These include being hearing impaired or blind, using a wheelchair, having severe asthma, a bad back, or chronic fatigue. Most disabilities are not passed genetically to unborn children. However, if you are planning on becoming pregnant, you may want to see a genetic counselor to discuss any risks that may be involved for you in pregnancy and for your children in inheriting your condition, whatever it may be. Make sure you find a midwife or doctor who believes in your ability to have a healthy pregnancy and childbirth and who will be honest but not condescending about any risks involved for you. It's imperative that you organize your house well beforehand and line up lots of extra support for after the baby's birth if you think you'll need it. If you can, plan on extra time to recover from your delivery and to get used to the demands of parenthood.

It's likely that there will be people who won't understand your desire to become pregnant, or who will assume that you will be unable to cope with a child once it's born. While it's not your job to educate everyone, you should be prepared during pregnancy for questions that will come your way concerning your disability. You may also find that many people express strong opinions about you even trying to become pregnant. The best form of support for disabled women may be talking with other disabled women who have successfully become pregnant and are parenting children. While local support groups may provide camaraderie, internet chat groups may be easier to participate in if you have a disability that keeps you closer to home.

The Weight Issue

> I was overweight by about fifty pounds when I got pregnant. The doctor didn't seem to think it would impede conception or cause undue stress during pregnancy or birth. I did not develop gestational diabetes, hypertension, or any other medical problem other than sciatica (leg pain radiating from the lower back). But I still advocate getting as much excess weight off as possible before getting pregnant, because complications can result. I was just extremely lucky!—Roberta

Many doctors will tell larger-sized women they need to lose weight before conceiving. It is true that obesity can lead to some health problems, and pregnancy certainly puts an extra strain and additional pounds on your body. So losing weight can make your pregnancy easier and help avoid complications. However, there is no real reason for most slightly or moderately overweight women to lose weight to conceive or bear children. If you are overweight but in good health and spirits, and you find that your doctor discourages your efforts to become pregnant, you may want to seek out a different health care practitioner. The best thing to remember is to be in the best shape that you can before getting pregnant. This holds true for women of all sizes.

Support System

If You Are Single

There is no doubt that it is hard to be a single mother. Proper planning will be absolutely necessary to set up a support system that works for you and your child once he or she arrives. While pregnant, you will need the support of both childless friends and other mamas to talk to and to help you get ready for the baby. Raising a child is often overwhelming, especially when you are alone with a small child for extended periods of time. The needs of babies are so intense that it can drive you nuts to give and give without a break. It is simply too much to expect that you can do it all by yourself, no matter how much you want a child. It's really a life saver to be able to call up a friend or designated "auntie" and be able to say "I'm losing it, please come over and take the baby for an hour." Having a friend relieve you for even a few hours a week can make a big difference in your emotional state.

The best time to start priming friends for becoming aunties is even before conception. Let friends know you are going to attempt to get pregnant. Talk to them about what this will mean for you, and ask them if they would like to participate in the baby's life. Some friends will be excited, others lukewarm to the idea, and still others clearly uninterested. But don't expect people's initial reactions to be set in stone. Many people will change their minds one way or another over the course of your pregnancy. I think if you can find even two or three people to provide ongoing auntie care for your growing child, you are doing well. This echoes my own experience, since out of a circle of about ten friends I'd hoped would participate in my baby's life, only three really became and remained involved. One or two I thought would especially want to be involved seemed to disappear into the drama of their own lives.

Keeping your eyes out for a trusted child care provider even before the baby's born will help you ease into a comfortable relationship with your first baby-sitter.

If You Are Coupled

If you are in a couple planning on raising a child together, you obviously have one another to count on during the pregnancy and after the baby arrives. However, babies are more work than you can plan on and may overwhelm even the best-prepared couples. Especially in the difficult early months, it is best to have established a support system of people who can at least help with cooking and cleaning. Luxuries like child care for an occasional meal out together will go far in maintaining some sanity in your lives and stability in your relationship. As the baby grows you will all benefit from having at least a few friends or family members involved in your child's life.

Health Tests You Will Need

Even before you start inseminating, eat like a queen, use only purified water, get in the habit of exercising regularly, and quit smoking. It really isn't too early to prepare the future baby-building machine for the most wholesome environment you can give that little one.—Stephanie

Allow two months before you actually start trying to get pregnant to have these tests and get the results. If you don't, you may be disappointed if the test process drags on and you can't begin trying to conceive right when you were planning to.

Now is the time to see what condition your body is in to grow a baby. While you may feel totally healthy and have no symptoms of illness, most fertility clinics and sperm banks will ask that you have a variety of health tests before you begin trying to conceive. It can be time- consuming and expensive to do so, but I suggest you get all the recommended tests. Typical tests you may be required to receive include both Pap and chlamydia smears, blood work for HIV, HTLV-1, CMV, syphilis, rubella, toxoplasmosis (see sidebar), Tay-Sachs (a fairly rare genetic disease

Toxoplasmosis

Toxoplasmosis is a disease that can cause birth defects in the baby if the mother is infected during pregnancy. It is contracted from the feces of cats who have eaten mice. If you already have the antibodies to toxoplasmosis before you are pregnant, you can't pass it on to your fetus. But if you test negative, you must be extremely careful changing your cat's litter box while you are pregnant. Have someone else do it or wear disposable rubber gloves each time you change the box. I kept a box of gloves on a table right next to the litter box so I wouldn't forget. Try to keep the box as clean as you can to avoid inhaling the fumes of feces.

among some Jews), and sickle-cell disease if you are African American. My sperm bank even insisted I receive a test for something called myco-ure-aplasma, which is a low-grade infection of the reproductive tract that many women have without realizing it. It is suspected of causing miscarriage and can prevent you from getting pregnant. I scoffed at taking that one in particular, and guess what—I tested positive for it. Luckily, a small dose of antibiotics cleared it from my system. Because of my experience, I would urge you to ask for this test even if your doctor doesn't require it. If you have a history of endometriosis, you may want to have a test to see if your fallopian tubes are viable. You may need laproscopic surgery to unblock the tubes and get rid of any adhesions or remaining endometriosis.

The Long and Winding Road Ahead

Despite all the stories you may have heard from other women about what it means to be pregnant or have a baby, your own experience will be completely different. For lesbians, getting pregnant is not so much a quick decision as a long and winding road fraught with detours, potholes, and the occasional stunning vista. Consider this woman's story:

My partner of fifteen years and I have been in the process of becoming moms for five years. We've been through her not want-

ing to be a mom, moving through that process, coming out to her parents about wanting to be moms, working with a known donor and developing a contract, meeting with a lawyer and two different counselors to make it work, that not working, advertising and meeting other potential known donors, working with a gay male couple and developing a contract, that not working, deciding to go the anonymous donor route, my losing my job, trying home-based insemination for six months, finding a job, going with an IUI in the doctor's office, getting pregnant, miscarrying at twelve weeks, not being able to get pregnant again, then going the infertility route with Clomid and facing the possibility of having my eggs harvested if it doesn't work this way! How did it get so complicated?—Sarah

Somehow, there's a lot more to this pregnancy stuff than meets the eye. You may decide that you aren't really ready to go through with all this yet. Or you may decide that you're not really sure you want to carry a baby and want to consider adoption instead. Or you may feel even more determined that you are ready to begin trying to get pregnant—immediately!

Only you can decide if you're ready to be a mother, and it's a big decision to make. For more reading on deciding whether to become a mom, I recommend Cheri Pies's *Considering Parenthood*. It is a bit outdated as a text but still an excellent first book to help you decide whether motherhood is really for you.

If you decide it is, you'll embark on a wondrous journey to bring a new baby into the world. Turn the page to begin...

2

Getting Started...
Now the Fun
Really Begins!

Now the fun begins! You've had all your health tests, you've probably thought about donor choices, and you're raring to start trying to get pregnant. But please read this chapter even if you think you just want to get started tomorrow on the whole process. The more you learn now, the smoother it will all go later. And you'll have also received a great education about how your body works—a wonderful prelude to all the changes you'll learn about during your pregnancy. Even if you find just a few pieces of information here that you end up using, it'll be worth it.

On Actually Trying to Get Pregnant

> *So many heterosexual pregnancies seem to happen by accident. But being a lesbian, I have spent years getting to this point. Thinking and wondering and thinking some more. And now the time has come to begin to try...—Iris*

If you're like many lesbians and have never been sexually active with men, fertility issues will be a brave new world to you! But even if you're like me and you spent your teenage years trying *not* to get pregnant with your male partners, you may not know a lot about how your body actually

you've never been pregnant, you may not even believe your body
e of becoming so. Now suddenly, after years of being with women
anu g...ng nary a thought to birth control, conception, or pregnancy, here
you are, wanting to get pregnant and maybe not knowing where to start.
It's frightening to start paying out lots of money not knowing if the
process will even work. But learning to trust in your body and knowing
how conception happens and how you can maximize your chances of it
happening is an empowering first step along the way to parenthood.

What Happens During Conception

The Mystery of Ovulation

Consider this your basic course in Conception 101. How does that one little sperm meet that ripe and ready egg, anyway? It's a miraculous process
worthy of sonnets, but we'll be brief and factual here. During each cycle,
if you are ovulating regularly, your body assumes pregnancy can occur.
Shortly after you finish your period, about fifteen eggs, each in its own fol-
licle, start to mature. One will eventually burst through the ovarian wall
while the rest disintegrate (unless multiple ovulation, responsible for multiple births, occurs). This process is called *ovulation,* and it usually happens
around the middle, or day 14, of a "typical" twenty-eight-day cycle.

If you want to get more detailed, know that the first half of your cycle
is called the *follicular phase.* This is the phase when your body is busy
preparing that next batch of eggs for fertilization. The follicles in which the
eggs are encased mature until that one lucky egg (or that egg and its com-
panions!) is released. What makes the whole thing difficult is trying to
determine *when* that egg will be ready, and therefore when to inseminate.
This is because the race to release an egg is one that varies in time from
woman to woman, and even from cycle to cycle in the same woman.

This follicular phase of your cycle lasts from the day you get your
period till ovulation, whenever that occurs. The amount of estrogen in
your body peaks at the point just before the egg is released, and this
surge of something called the *luteinizing hormone* is what the ovulation
predictor kits monitor. That is why usually you will inseminate a day or
so *after* you see that you have "surged."

The second phase of your cycle, which is called the *luteal phase,* lasts from ovulation to the last day before the start of your next period. This is usually about twelve to sixteen days in length. That is why when you are learning to track ovulation, a more accurate way of judging your timing is to know that it occurs about fourteen days *before* the start of your *next* period. Of course, although many books and doctors talk about the typical twenty-eight-day cycle, a good percentage of women do not have twenty-eight-day cycles! Anywhere from twenty- to forty-day cycles are normal, with some women menstruating only once every several months. You can see how this changes how you judge when ovulation takes place.

Once the egg bursts through the ovarian wall, it will get sucked up, often in less than half an hour, by the nearby fallopian tube and stay alive for between six to twenty-four hours, awaiting fertilization. If conception is going to happen, it is most often because sperm are already there in the outer fallopian tube, waiting for it. Sperm freshly ejaculated can survive for up to five days inside a woman (although three days is more common), and women who use fresh sperm therefore have a larger window of time in which sperm can meet egg. Thus, women who inseminate with fresh sperm usually get pregnant much sooner.

Remember that even under the best of circumstances, conception does not always occur!

The shorter life span for frozen sperm of about one to two days means that timing becomes absolutely critical. Inseminating at home with frozen sperm generally means that the sperm must make an arduous journey through the fertile cervical mucus, up through the vagina, into the cervix, and toward the egg. This can take about five hours. Out of the life span of twenty-four hours, this is a big chunk of time, and there's a lot less time to hang around in there or find the egg. A process called an *intrauterine insemination* (more details on that in a minute!) cuts down on the travel time of the sperm by placing them right in the cervix or uterus, rather than in the vagina.

If Sperm Meets Egg

If a sperm does meet the egg, it's generally one of the most hardy and best swimmers. With the help of other sperm that are also trying, it penetrates the egg. Fertilization has occurred! But conception has a few more steps to it. First, this newly fertilized egg tumbles through the fallopian tube, ever dividing, till after a few days it enters the uterus. It is producing increasing amounts of hCG (human Chorionic Gonadotrophin), a hormone that pregnancy tests measure for and that can be detected about two weeks later. After a few more days in the uterus, this ball of cells—called a blastocyst—contains about a hundred cells and is ready to burrow into the uterine lining. If it successfully embeds itself, implantation has occurred, and it will grow here for the next nine months.

If conception does not occur, the uterine lining will soon be shed (often with the tiny egg in it) and you will menstruate. Then the whole cycle repeats itself all over again.

RECOMMENDED READING

Beginning Life: The Marvelous Journey from Conception to Birth by Geraldine Lux Flanagan features incredible, highly magnified color pictures of the conception process.

Can You Plan for a Boy or Girl?

It seems that more lesbians want to have girl children than boy children. Of course, it is the father's sperm that determines whether you have a boy or girl child. The common wisdom is that alternative insemination produces more boys. This does seem particularly true when using frozen sperm. One factor that probably contributes to this is that most women inseminate only once or twice a cycle when they use frozen sperm, as close to the time of ovulation as possible. Because boy sperm (which carry the Y chromosome) are thought to swim faster but die faster, they have an advantage over the hardier, slower-swimming girl sperm (which carry the X chromosome). Those boy sperm just dart up there and grab the egg before the girl sperm have a chance. If you were inseminating a few days before ovulation, the girl sperm could hang out and wait for the egg, outliving the boy sperm. The problem is that if you use the frozen goods, none of it can live that long. You really just have a window of a day or two of peak fertility to inseminate when using frozen sperm.

However, fresh sperm does live longer than a day or two. Sometimes, it can live up to a week! So *theoretically*, using fresh sperm, particularly over the course of the week leading up to ovulation, will probably increase your odds of having a girl. And most lesbians using frozen sperm will probably have boys.

In the end, this is all just speculation. Several friends of mine used live donors and had boys. I used frozen sperm the morning after I ovulated and had a girl. New theories prove one thing, then another theory disproves the last one. There is just no way to tell which sex your child will be, even if you use one of the high-tech (and expensive) sperm-sorting methods currently becoming available. One day there may be a cheap, affordable way to make sex selection more accessible and dependable. Till then, you have to take what you get!

Checking Your Fertility

To any woman starting to try to get pregnant, I would say, read and learn about your own fertility. Once you really begin this process, you will be better able to advocate for yourself.—Joyce

Because as a lesbian you generally have only one or two tries each month to attempt to become pregnant, it is imperative that you learn how to tell if and when you're fertile. This is not hard to do, and soon you will become an expert at it.

There are several ways you can check to tell when you are most fertile. It will take a cycle or two to become familiar with them and decide which methods you will use as conception tools.

Cervical Mucus

Once I began tracking my fertile mucus, I realized just what this goo I had always noticed actually was! It was a great indicator of when I was about to ovulate. It was like, here comes the mucus, phone up the sperm bank!—Natalie

One of the most reliable fertility signs is cervical mucus. Even if you think you don't know a thing about it, you actually have probably been vaguely aware of its presence. Have you ever noticed white stains in your underwear, or gooey stuff appearing on the toilet paper you've used? What you've seen is cervical mucus, but you've probably just taken it in stride as a regular bodily function and not thought to question its varying appearances. But cervical mucus holds a giant part of the key to conception. Therefore, it warrants closer inspection here.

Cervical mucus is produced by all ovulating women. The quantity and consistency will vary from woman to woman, cycle to cycle, and day to day. Your mucus can be affected by the weather, or even by the stress of trying to conceive, so even within individual women, each cycle will be different. And some women never produce much, in which case this will not be the most useful fertility sign

If you have a partner, and you both want her to get involved, you can put her in charge of fertility checks and charts. She can be the one to read the pee sticks, check your cervical position, and analyze your mucus. She can be in charge of temperature-taking and maintaining your temperature chart. This will help her feel involved even though you're the one whose body this all depends on!

to track. Still, it is amazing how much the variations of your mucus have to do with how you get pregnant.

Here are the phases that a typical woman's mucus goes through:

During your period, you will not notice much mucus, because you are bleeding—but get ready for the changes soon afterward.

In the days right after your period, you will find that you either have no mucus or are very dry at your vaginal opening. There probably won't be any show in your underpants at this point.

After a few days, you may begin to get what is called "sticky" mucus. It can be rubbery looking, or kind of clumpy, but not very wet or gooey. You are not yet fertile.

Next, your mucus may become creamy, looking somewhat like hand lotion. It may put a spot in your underwear. You are getting fertile at this point.

Now you will probably be close to the midpoint of your cycle, ready for the appearance of fertile mucus. It will be very different from the creamy stuff of a few days before. It will probably be fairly clear (or have a slight yellow tinge), and it may have a stretchy quality like that of egg whites. If you put some between your fingers it should stretch out at least an inch, if not up to several inches in length. This stretchiness is called *spinnbarkeit*; we will call it *spin* for short. It may sound odd at first, but soon you will be asking yourself, "Am I spinny yet?" since spin is one of the best indicators of fertility.

I would recommend beginning to learn about your mucus right after you finish a period. This will allow you to track a cycle from beginning to end.

So What About Spin?

Why should you care about spin, and what does it do for you?

If you were to look at different kinds of cervical fluid under a microscope, you would see that mucus acts very much like a barrier to sperm for most of your cycle. It's like a tangled web that sperm gets caught in.

When you get spin (or fertile mucus), it's as if the channel doors opened. Suddenly, there are pathways for the sperm to swim through into your cervix on the way to meet the egg. It's as if our bodies have a defense mechanism against letting sperm through before the egg is ready.

Once your body lets you know that ovulation is beckoning by producing spin, your window of opportunity narrows. If you are in your twenties or early thirties, you may get spin for several days, but if you are older, you may notice it only for a day or so. There are various remedies women can try to produce more fertile mucus, including downing Robitussin cough syrup (an expectorant that seems to thin the cervical mucus, making it easier for sperm to pass through) and drinking horrible-tasting Chinese teas. I tried a concoction we got in Chinatown and became spinny beyond belief. Some women who ordinarily may be a bit dehydrated (perhaps from drinking too much coffee and caffeinated soft drinks) may also find that simply drinking more water will help them produce more mucus, especially in the hot summer months.

After ovulation happens, your spin dries up quickly, and you will be fairly dry for the rest of your cycle. You are no longer fertile.

Other Kinds of Mucus

Sometimes you hear reports about women who produce "hostile mucus," and for them it's even harder to conceive, as their mucus does not seem to want to allow sperm in at all. Or it may just kill the sperm on contact! While it may seem like a humorous idea that lesbians could have sperm-killing mucus, for women trying to conceive it is maddening. You can only really find out if this is the case by taking a sample of your vaginal fluid right after an insemination. If the sperm are dead, you know you've got a problem! Talk to your doctor about how best to remedy this in your particular situation.

VAGINAL INFECTIONS. If you have any strange- or bad-smelling discharge or suspect you have a yeast or vaginal infection, get this checked out and cleared up at least a month before starting to try to conceive.

AROUSAL FLUID. The fluid your body produces when you're sexually excited is *not* the same as fertile mucus!

LUBRICANTS. If you are expecting to inseminate within a day or two, it's best to avoid heavy use of lube during sex play. According to Cathy Winks and Anne Semans, authors of *The New Good Vibrations Guide to Sex*, the "preservative ingredients" in all lubes "are capable of killing sperm"—even in water-based lubes not containing nonoxynol-9. Of course you will not want to use any lubricant or lubricated condoms containing nonoxynol-9, a detergent that has been shown in some laboratory experiments to reduce the rate of HIV transmission by killing the HIV virus. Nonoxynol-9 also kills sperm. Check the fine print on the package. The last thing you want to realize the day you're about to inseminate is that you used a spermicide the night before! Oops!

Things That Might Affect Your Fertility

Some women have minor or even serious health problems that may curtail their ability to get pregnant. These include endometriosis, pelvic inflammatory disease, and fibroids. You should consult a doctor if you have previously suffered from any such conditions or if you have ever had surgery on any part of your reproductive tract. Before you jump on the conception roller coaster, it's good to know what your chances are of becoming pregnant, and how to maximize your odds.

However, there are a number of common-sense things that any woman can do to boost her everyday odds of getting pregnant. These include avoiding radiation, toxins, including those in paints, and overexposure to computer monitors. You should also cut back on caffeine and alcohol, both of which have been proven to affect fertility. Some people also believe that hot-tubbing may damage your eggs. Douching is also a poor idea, since it changes the pH balance of your vagina, the last thing you want to be doing right now! Overexercising or dieting may also impede conception, as will stress. And since stress is certainly going to be part of your life from now on, it's best to find ways to minimize it where you can. For more on stress relief, see chapter 4, "Surviving the Roller Coaster." To naturally improve their fertility, many women turn to acupuncture, special teas, and meditation.

Taking Your Temperature

*After you've been doing this for a while, you may wish for a
morning where you can just bound out of bed without taking
your temperature. Just check for a month every now and then so
you don't burn out on it.—Ava*

Taking your temperature every morning is like boot camp for fertility
awareness. Exciting for one cycle, obsessive for a few more, then merely
annoying, till you just want to throw the thermometer across the room.
And your girlfriend may well do just that after being awakened every
morning by that little beep-beep at 7:00 A.M. Rather than an everyday
thermometer, you need to use a special basal body thermometer, which
measures tenths of degrees within the 95- to 99-degree range. These are
available in most drugstores for under $20. I like the digital ones for their
ease of use though some clinics recommend only the mercury variety,
which may be more accurate. Before you ovulate, your temperature is
low, but a surge of progesterone in your body after ovulation causes your
temperature to rise. If you get pregnant, your temperature will stay high
(or even rise higher). If you're not, it will generally fall dramatically the
day before or the day you actually bleed. This lets you know your period
is coming—which is, of course, quite upsetting when you're trying to get
pregnant! It's best to take your temperature first thing in the morning,
before you move around at all, to get a more accurate reading. Charting
your cycle a few times will bring you in tune with what these slight but
important variations in temperature will mean for you, and you will begin
to notice a distinct pattern to your body's temperature. This is also a surefire way of determining if indeed you are even ovulating, a good thing to
know before you start the rest of this whole process.

How it all works: You will fill out a chart marking your waking temperature before you even roll out of bed to pee. Each day you'll place a
dot on the chart to record your temperature. Connect the dots and you
will see the natural rhythm of your body. Start each chart with your
period. Note the dates of your spin and the date of your surge. It will typically look something like this, although please remember that every
woman's cycle length is different. You'll find a blank chart in the
Appendix; feel free to make copies.

Basal Body Temperature Chart April ~ May '99

insemination by IUI

Days of Cycle	1	2	3	4	5	6	7	8	9	10	11	12	13	14	15	16	17	18	19	20	21	22	23	24	25	26	27	28	29	30	31	32	33	34	35	36	37	38	39	40	41	42
Date of Month	26	27	28	29	30	1	2	3	4	5	6	7	8	9	10	11	12	13	14	15	16	17	18	19	20	21	22	23	24	25	26											
Spin																		X	X	X	X																					
Surge												sticky	sticky	sticky	sticky	creamy	creamy		S		K-P 97.45	K-P									X											
Menstruation	X	X	X	X																																						

I have to warn you that charting your periods can make you terribly obsessive, and if you're like me, the stress of trying to get pregnant will cause your cycles, and therefore your charts, to veer all over the place. After about four tries, I didn't chart my periods anymore except to note when I had spin, when I surged, the day I inseminated, and when I bled. Other women find charting their cycles to be a comforting process. I think for the first month or two it's a useful tool, but if the charts start annoying you, don't worry about completing them. Some sperm banks and clinics want you to fill one out every month. But hey, it's your body and your money, so do what works for you.

Try charting the different phases of mucus on your temperature chart and you will begin to see how your fertility signs all work together!

Also, please note that while ovulation kits (see below) have become the most popular way of determining the time of insemination, only by taking your temperature will you know if you have actually released an egg.

Ovulation Kits

One of the easiest and most convenient methods of testing for your ovulation is with what are officially called *ovulation predictor kits,* or less formally, "pee sticks." There are several brands commercially available in most large drugstores, although you may have to ask for them at the pharmacy counter. Generally, the kits cost about $20–$25 for a one-month supply, but you may be able to stretch them over two cycles once you get the hang of your ovulation cycle.

Ovulation kits are small plastic strips about five inches long. They have a place to pee on one end and a window on the other end for results. You pee on one end of the thing for a few seconds, then you flip it over, wait a few seconds, and watch for a reading that you can compare to the "test" line in the window. Usually, you will do this test around noon, after holding your urine for a few hours. This is so your hormonal levels can build up in your pee. Your first morning pee is not recommended since it often won't indicate you are surging, even if you are. Make *sure* you read the instructions that come with each different type of kit you buy.

What the test measures is the LH or luteinizing hormone, which appears in your urine most strongly right before ovulation. This is formally called your *surge*. It means that you are about to ovulate within twelve to twenty-four hours. If you test and no line appears, you are not about to ovulate, or you have already ovulated. If a faint line appears, ovulation is still a few days away, and you should keep testing until the line is equal to or darker than the test line. You will be waiting for that maximum dark blue line to appear before you take any action. In general, the darker the line appears, the closer you are to ovulation. If you have two days where the test line appears to be equally dark, you have probably caught the surge as it rises and falls. This may be especially true if you test twice a day and see a surge at night and again the following morning.

Make sure you stock up on or order ovulation kits well in advance of when you may need them! The last thing you want is to have a miss a month because you ran out of kits.

The tricky part of this is that some of the commercially available tests, like Clearplan Easy, may not show a line that ever gets very dark or darker than the test line, which is what you are hoping for. A better, though more expensive test kit is called Ovu-Quick. I recommend their One-Step 6 Day Test Kit over the Four-Step, as it is almost as easy to use as the Clearplan Easy test and much more accurate. Ovu-Quick products are worth the extra cost. However, you will probably need to mail order the kits as opposed to buying them in a local drugstore. One box costs about $25 plus shipping. You can call Conception Technologies at (800) 995-8081 and charge the kits to a credit card.

Whatever kind of kit you initially try, don't be afraid to try a different kind the following month. Different kits work better for different women. And remember that it is best to also check for other signs of fertility as a backup.

One other thing to know is that some fertility drugs may render these tests invalid. Clomid, however, is not thought to have this effect.

More About the Surge

Although some women notice a surge on only one day, some women find that they surge for two or more days, and are therefore unsure which days are best for insemination. Generally, the kits tell you to consider the first day of the strongest signs of a surge your peak day. It's important to remember that the surge tells you that you will ovulate within a day or two, not that you are ovulating right then. Thus, if you inseminate too early, frozen sperm, which are less hardy than the fresh variety, may die before the egg is available for fertilization. You need to be as accurate as possible in determining your surge, then wait twenty-four hours—and this part of the process is very frustrating! My inclination was always to try as soon as the surge stick turned blue, which was probably too early. It is more than a bit tricky to know what the perfect time is each cycle until after it passes, so there may be some months when you miss the moment. Obviously, the more times you can inseminate each cycle, the better your luck will be. It's easy to get into a tizzy about what your optimum day is, especially when you are having intrauterines done at a clinic and can afford only one try a month. Some women try right at their peak, others wait a day, some even two, while others like to inseminate a day before they peak on their surge, in part to better the odds of having a girl. The time I actually got pregnant I was convinced I'd waited too long, as it was a day or so after the peak of my surge, my cervix was partially closed, and I was sure I had already ovulated. I had little hope that the egg would be able to live that long. As it turns out, I was either extremely lucky or I had been inseminating too early on previous tries. In any case, relying just on the pee sticks to predict ovulation is not as effective as combining their results with other fertility signs. Still, for many women, because of their ease of use, pee sticks remain the primary way of deciding what day to inseminate.

Other Fertility Signs

Most of these additional fertility signs are unnecessary to check for unless you're really a stickler for details. They include the angle of your cervix (which I never really could see or figure out), which will sit higher and feel softer when you're fertile. Some women check under a microscope for their cervical mucus to appear fern-like, guaranteeing that the sperm can swim through it, and some women regularly feel their egg burst through the ovarian wall at the height of their fertility. This is called *mittelschmerz* (midpain) and will most often be felt just on one side of your body, sometimes for up to a few hours. I would feel it and think, "Ouch, I have gas!" then realize what it actually was.

Another sign to check for is the degree of openness of your cervix. This will bear close inspection, particularly if you're using a speculum during your insemination. Normally, your cervix appears closed, but as you get to your peak time of fertility, it will gradually become open, and you may see it covered in or oozing fertile mucus. If your cervix is really wide open, this is a good indication that your body

RECOMMENDED READING

Taking Charge of Your Fertility *by Toni Weschler. Although the book has a heterosexual focus and the author talks a lot about "when to have sex with your husband," her focus on every fertility sign and lengthy explanation of fertile mucus— complete with pictures—as well as her reassuring tone make this book a good investment.*

is inviting those little sperm to swim right on in there and go for it! I always asked whomever was doing my insemination about the degree to which my cervix was open. And if it was closed, I had a pretty good idea that the insemination wasn't going to work, since ovulation either had not yet occurred or had already passed. Ideally, you could check openness at home before going to the clinic, but if you don't have a speculum, or if you just hate poking around up there, you may not want to check this yourself.

Some women will also feel increasingly sexual as their ovulation approaches. It's as if nature were letting you know that now is the time to try! Personally, I have never felt so lushly sexual in my life as when I began trying to get pregnant and knew ovulation was near.

Other "secondary" fertility signs may include a bit of spotting, water retention, and breast tenderness. You may have always experienced some small degree of many of these signs but never noticed them or thought to associate them with anything in particular. But believe me, by the time you have tried to get pregnant at least a few times, you will know them all, and all too well!

Getting the Goods

Sperm: The Necessary Ingredient

Sperm. It's a substance many of us have shied away from most of our lives. But now that you've made the decision to get pregnant, it's a necessity. How do you get it? What do you do with it once you have it? This chapter will explore how to obtain sperm, how much it'll cost you, and how to protect yourself legally in the process.

Sperm Versus Semen

When a man ejaculates, the fluid he produces is called semen. In this fluid usually swim millions of sperm. Every man produces different quantities of live and healthy sperm, which is measured as his "sperm count." When you use freshly ejaculated semen, or the frozen stuff from the sperm bank, you are inseminating with sperm that are still in the semen. However, if you go to a clinic for a procedure such as an intrauterine, where the sperm are fed more directly into the vagina, most often you are being inseminated only with sperm. This is because the clinic has already spun the slower swimmers and any that may be dead out of the semen for higher effectiveness. In this book, I'll talk primarily about sperm, as opposed to semen, since it is the sperm that actually causes you to get pregnant.

Known Versus Unknown Donor: The Big Decision

One of the biggest decisions you will make in trying to get pregnant is whether to use a known or an unknown donor. It should be a decision on which you spend some time. Don't rush into the first available option just because you want to get started. How you create your child will have long-lasting implications on your life, so it's best to consider all the issues involved. You should take special care to thoroughly examine the legal implications involved if you want to use a known donor.

Using a Known Donor

There are many reasons why women may choose to use a known donor:
- You know what the donor looks like and acts like.
- You will theoretically be able to try inseminating more than once a cycle, bettering your chances of conceiving sooner.
- Fresh sperm is more active and therefore, you may conceive sooner.
- Your child can have a relationship with the donor as he or she grows up.
- You have a male friend who really wants to help out.
- You can use a gay man as your donor, whereas most sperm banks will only use heterosexuals as donors.
- You think you cannot afford to use frozen sperm.
- The donor may be genetically linked to the nonbiological mother in a couple (it could be her brother, perhaps), thereby guaranteeing her some biological connection to the child.
- You feel you have no access to a sperm bank or clinic that meets your needs.

Of course, you may think you have the perfect male specimen in mind, but when you ask him to donate, he says no. Or he might tell you that he has HIV or some other disease. Or he might initially agree, then back out. You will have to see how it goes—and don't be devastated if the "perfect" donor doesn't work out. Whoever your donor ends up being, your baby will likely still be the "perfect" baby for you.

Some Things to Know
About Using Fresh Donor Sperm

The most usual scenario for donating fresh sperm is for the donor to come over, masturbate in the bathroom, and ejaculate into a container. Then he usually presents his semen and leaves, letting the woman or women get on with the insemination.

Sperm should be collected from the donor in a cup or bowl that is clean, at room temperature, and made of glass or plastic.

The collected sperm should be kept at body temperature until used. Sometimes you may need to transport the sperm from one location to another. In this case, you should keep the receptacle containing the sperm as close to your body as possible to keep it warm.

Fresh sperm can live up to a few hours once ejaculated, but it is best to use it immediately, or at least within an hour.

To the lesbian eye, the quantity of semen in a single ejaculate may look rather small. As long as there is enough to fill a needless syringe, you have more than enough to try and get pregnant!

I initially wanted to use a known donor, but I changed my mind after three separate men had to come out to me as HIV-positive when I asked them. One even said he'd considered lying to me about his status because he wanted a child so badly. That scared me enough to only consider using a sperm bank from then on.—Theresa

We had a close friend who took an AIDS test. He came over three days in a row and did his donation in a sterile dish. We did not consult any doctors, nor did we use any drugs. The donor sees our son every so often but does not want to be a significant part of his life. He knew right from the beginning that it was "right" to donate to us.—Patrice

Asking a Guy to Be Your Donor

Sometimes the right man will be in your life before you even decide to get pregnant. You'll ask him, he'll say yes, you'll inseminate, and then you'll get pregnant. Wow! That sounds easy, and for some women it is. More typical, however, is the experience of having to scout around for a while. After thinking about what you are looking for in a donor, you will have to decide if anyone you know fits the bill. If they don't, you will have to continue looking.

How do you find a donor? My friend Andrea once stopped a guy at a crosswalk and asked him. He was cute and she liked his look. That might be a little extreme, but it's not entirely off track. A good donor can be almost anywhere. He could be your partner's gay cousin, or an old dear straight friend who's already married with children. He could even be the guy who serves you your morning chai. The trick is to find someone whose health is good, who will actually work with you on this (because it will be work for him too!), and whom you can talk with and trust.

Unfortunately, finding the right guy can take a while. If you try to rush things with a man, the fit may not be good, and it won't work out for anyone involved. If you feel that you aren't finding the right person, take a breather. You might need to take a wider look around at your circle of friends and acquaintances. Ask your friends if they know any great guys who might be interested in helping you out. Make sure people know that you are looking and that you're ready to start.

Things to Think About When Using a Known Donor

YOU MUST SCREEN THE DONOR'S HEALTH YOURSELF.
This means the onus is on you, for your health and the health of your baby, to make sure the donor is healthy. Many men will agree to be a donor but balk at taking a battery of medical tests (which you will likely

When you do approach a man about being a donor, don't ask questions like "Have you always wanted to be a father?" This will give the wrong impression about the role you actually expect him to play. You might start by saying, "You know, I've been [or "we've been," if you're in a couple] giving a lot of thought to having a baby. I'm looking for a man to donate his sperm to me to help me get pregnant. Is that something you'd ever be interested in?" Keep things light during the first conversation about it. Make sure you're clear that this is not about sex and that you're only looking for a sperm donation. Make sure he understands he will not be considered the father (if this is the case), and that he has to be okay with that. Suggest that he think about it for a week and that you talk in more detail about things then. You'll most likely hear a definite no or maybe. Most guys will want to ponder what this would mean to them before they commit. That's probably a good thing. You haven't made your decision lightly to ask him, so you'll want him to respond in kind. If he says yes right away, suggest he take that week to think things through anyway.

When you meet again, if he says yes, proceed with caution through the next phase of negotiations. If he says no, move on. There is no point in trying to cajole someone to get him to change his mind, as this could cause problems later. If he still is saying maybe, decide with him when you can expect to have a firm answer. If he doesn't give you an answer by then, move on. Some guys will keep you hanging for a while if you let them. Consider that kind of response a no and look for someone else.

have to pay for if he's uninsured). You should screen your donor for the same conditions screened by any quality sperm bank: HIV, syphilis, hepatitis B and C, HTLV 1, cytomegalovirus (CMV), gonorrhea, chlamydia, myco-ureaplasma, complete blood count, liver and kidney function, past medical history, family medical history, and blood type.

YOU WILL HAVE TO TRUST HIS BEHAVIOR IMPLICITLY.
This includes trusting that over the time you spend trying to get pregnant (whether that be a month or three years), he will engage only in safer-sex activities, curtail his consumption of drugs and alcohol, wear loose underwear, and avoid hot tubs to keep his sperm count up.

Will you be comfortable talking with your donor about sex? Whether his sperm enters your body via a syringe or through passionate sex, you still have to negotiate what you mean by "safer sex." Some men define it as using a condom for anal intercourse—but may engage in other sex play without a latex barrier. Some practices that are effective in preventing HIV are not so effective in preventing other STDs, such as herpes.

You can find information on safer-sex practices for men from your local AIDS service organization or online from the Stop AIDS Project (www.stopaids.org) or The Safer Sex Pages (www.safersex.org).

HE MAY NOT BE AVAILABLE WHEN YOU ARE OVULATING.
Let's face it—people lead busy lives. Even men who give this a great deal of thought may find that they do not want to be on call 24/7. If they have to travel for business, or are impulsive in recreational travel, you may find you are missing chances to inseminate. This can become extremely frustrating.

The Legal Experts Speak on Known Donors

> Using a known donor is a minefield of risk.—Kate Kendall, director, National Center for Lesbian Rights

Basically, unless a doctor is involved in both the exchange of sperm between donor and recipient and the insemination, using a known donor's fresh semen is not legally sound. The National Center for Lesbian Rights is very clear about this. In a publication called *Lesbians Choosing Motherhood: Legal Implications of Alternative Insemination and Reproductive Technologies*, they state, "By using a known donor without the supervision of a physician, you heighten the risk of being forced by the courts into an unwanted and unexpected parenting relationship with the donor." While a known donor may have the best of intentions, he may develop paternal feelings upon the birth of the child and may wish to be treated as a father.

Writes the NCLR, "While it is true that there are many roles that a donor can assume that fall somewhere between being a donor in name alone, and being a full-fledged father, it is important to recognize that in our system of law there are only two options. Either the donor is merely a donor, with no parental rights or relationship with the child whatsoever, or he is the father, with all his parental rights intact. There is no gray area in the law, and, when in doubt, the courts will grant donors full parental rights in cases involving single mothers."

NCLR director Kate Kendall says, "In concept, using a known donor is a great idea. It's the legal system that's the problem. Because unfortunately, if he sues for paternity, even in the face of an agreement [between donor and the mother], that agreement may be invalidated." Kendall concurs that using a known donor can work, but she urges women to remember to take their time when deciding on a man and to be prepared to walk away from the situation if red flags come up in preconception negotiations. "There is no other relationship that is so responsibility-filled and pervasive as being a parent. Don't choose a known donor like you'd choose a roommate."

> My advice is to use a sperm bank rather than a known donor. Your donor, although he may sign away his rights, could come back and sue for paternity. A judge could reverse any agreement and reinstate his parental rights, granting him visitation and possibly joint custody. Don't doubt that this couldn't happen to you. This is exactly what happened to us. It is not necessarily cheaper to use a known donor as opposed to a sperm bank. If a court case were to ensue it could run into thousands of dollars.—Wren

Now that I've scared you, let me also add that most known donor arrangements work out just fine. Kendall says that only about 10 percent of donor arrangements end up in litigation. For couples who know the donor well and have discussed every possible aspect of conflict in advance, it can be a rewarding experience for everyone involved. Many women I know have had good experiences using a known donor. A good friend of mine just got pregnant with baby number two from her donor, and the donor is a valued addition to their family. Other women use brothers of their partners, with nary a legal complication. Preparation and trust are essential, and sometimes taking a chance seems like the only way you'll get your baby. It can also be a more humane and even humorous way to conceive than the sterile methods employed at a clinic:

> In the first month I tried to get pregnant I ovulated early. I called my donor to see if he could make an impromptu donation. Our donor was at work, but he took a break and came up with the goods, which were then promptly delivered to our house by his partner. My girlfriend took one look at the specimen and asked "Is that all there is?" and our donor's partner got a little defensive, saying, "Well, he was a little stressed!" The things committed donors go through!—Jackie

> The first time we inseminated, we used a known donor and went to his house. My training as a counselor helped me listen both to the donor and to my partner as they expressed their feelings about their fears and apprehension over the unusual circumstances of what we were doing. I talked to the donor about the gift he was giving us and told him we could never forget this. But I had been with very few men before coming out, and the minute I looked into the cup that held his semen, I felt nauseated. The more nauseated I became, the more inept I became at managing the whole process. The turkey baster we had was entirely too big. I could not draw any sperm up into it but was only able to blow bubbles into the semen. I finally swallowed hard, put some on my finger…and literally took the plunge. The next day, we bought a 10cc syringe, and the rest of our inseminations went great!—Pam

> I'm white and my partner is Japanese American. When we decided that I would get pregnant, we asked her cousin to be our donor. That way we'd have a biracial child, and she could be related to the baby, too. We had legal papers drawn up but have never needed them. The donor, who lives in another city, acts as an "uncle" and sees our daughter a few times a year. It's been wonderful for all of us to see her grow up.—Hettie

When my son was four weeks old, his father took him two days a week for about three hours at a time. At nineteen months my son spent the night for the first time at his father's house. Most recently, his father spends two nights a week at our house, since he now lives a few hours away. All in all, it's an arrangement that's worked well for us.—Lara

See the Sample Donor-Recipient Agreement in the Appendix. This form, prepared by the NCLR, is a good first step in preparing documentation to use with a known donor. Like any legal document, though, it should be tailored to your own personal situation and state or provincial law by an attorney.

The Father Factor

I met him through a support group for prospective gay and lesbian parents. We only knew each other for four months before we decided we'd like to coparent a child. We spent a lot of time together talking about all the issues involved and worked out a parenting agreement, which we have never had to refer to. I got pregnant the second time we tried. Our daughter splits the time between his house and mine. We have been extremely lucky that we get along so well, and we always tell people that we don't recommend doing things as quickly as we did!—Theresa

There is another choice besides using the services of a sperm bank or a donor friend to get pregnant. Certainly it is not an option that legal experts would consider sound. Yet, for many women, it makes the most sense. And that is for the man with whom you became pregnant to be involved as a father in your child's life.

There are many women who find the idea of raising a child without a father less than desirable. The lesbian party line does not tend to favor this view, and there is much more support today for women using anonymous donors. Still, the concept of a donor is not for everyone. Some lesbians and bisexual women really want to have an involved father in their children's lives. They may also want the financial and emotional support that men can bring into the equation, as well as the opportunity to share parenting responsibilities. Some single women may prefer to coparent with a man rather than wait for the perfect female companion to come along. And some lesbian couples may have a longtime gay male couple with whom coparenting seems the natural choice in creating an extended family of parents to shower a child with love.

Indeed, there are many men, both straight and gay, who are looking for a way to father without having to parent full time. Some may be actively searching for a woman with whom to share parenting through a prospective gay parents group (see Resources for suggestions). Check your local gay/lesbian magazines for such a group, look for listings on the Internet, or even start your own group. Other men may not even have considered parenting as an option until they are approached by a woman friend or couple.

Just as there are many of us who seek a lesbian family relationship typical in structure to the stereotypical nuclear family, there are also many who are looking for ways to build a new family dynamic. This could include a family with two moms and two gay dads, a lesbian and a gay man coparenting together, a single lesbian coparenting with a gay male couple, a straight woman coparenting with a gay man, and a lesbian or bisexual woman co-parenting with a straight man. The woman who is the biological parent may receive the sperm in "donation" form or may actually have sex with the man who will be the biological father. The father may or may not be listed on the birth certificate, depending on the wishes of all involved.

There are certainly legal issues that must be addressed in any of these family setups. It is best, from a legal standpoint, not to leave issues of custody pending till after the baby's born. If you are considering a coparenting arrangement in any capacity with the man who will be your baby's father, make sure you know each other really well, and do your legal homework. Many wonderful families have been born this way.

Using a Sperm Bank

If you've decided you want to use a sperm bank, how do you begin to find one? There are more banks in the United States and Canada all the time. In other parts of the world you will have a harder time finding a

sperm bank, and even if you do, there may be no way they will inseminate a "single" woman. Certain states in the United States may also have
laws that prohibit sperm banks from sending deliveries to any place other
than a doctor's office. And those doctors may not be allowed to hand
over the sperm to let you do home inseminations, or may require paperwork from the sperm banks that states it is okay for them to do so. It's
really rather ridiculous that there are such restrictive policies about
sperm, but we can hope that these laws will change soon.

Certainly, legally and healthwise you are most protected by using
sperm from a sperm bank. Not only is the donor tested repeatedly for
diseases like HIV, but you can also be assured that his sperm mobility is
good, and in many cases he has already produced other live children. It
is also reassuring to know that the donor can never come after you for
custody, since he has legally signed his rights away.

Of the sperm banks in North America, some are geared more toward
straight couples experiencing fertility issues, while others were founded
expressly for single women and lesbians. Most now don't care so much
one way or another who their clients are. Word of mouth is probably the
best way to decide which bank you'll be most comfortable using. After
all, if friends of yours were treated well, you probably will be too. If you
don't know any women using sperm banks, my recommendation is to
contact some of the banks in this book's Resources section, send for their
information, and see what appeals to you.

Questions to Ask of a Sperm Bank

There are several basic questions you will need answered before you
decide on a sperm bank:

HOW "OUT" CAN YOU BE ABOUT YOUR LIFE?

If the sperm bank assumes its clientele is straight and acts accordingly,
you may have to do some educating, especially if you have an involved
partner who comes to all your appointments. On the other hand, you
may just be the bank's or clinic's first out lesbian couple, and they'll
adjust accordingly. With the "gay-by boom" raging on, you certainly
won't be their last! However, if the bank or clinic is just downright hostile to the idea of inseminating lesbians, look elsewhere. With the ability

to ship sperm from several lesbian-friendly banks across the United States direct to your living room, there's no reason to face homophobia where you don't have to. See the Resources chapter for the best lesbian-friendly sperm banks.

Words of Advice from Maura Riordan,
Director of the The Sperm Bank of California

Preparing for insemination can be very stressful. It's critical that women find the sperm bank that feels like the "right fit" for their needs. The importance of feeling a sense of control over the process and knowing that the sperm bank you're using is not just a business, but a supportive environment, cannot be underestimated. Fortunately, times are changing, and the sperm-banking industry is much less homophobic than it once was, but there are still a number of banks that aren't accustomed to working with lesbians and may use language (and make assumptions) based on heterosexual bias. It's important to shop around for the right sperm bank, which includes being open to the possibility of working with a bank in another state. Currently, sperm banks in urban areas such as San Francisco, Boston, and New York are most likely to work regularly with single women and lesbian couples and are better equipped to make the experience a positive and supportive one. The bottom line is that lesbians can and should expect to be treated respectfully and welcomed warmly by whatever bank they use.

HOW MANY DONORS DO YOU HAVE?
HOW MANY ARE ACTUALLY AVAILABLE?
There is an important difference here. One sperm bank I tried had about twenty to twenty-five active donors on record, but many of the more "desirable" donors were simply not available for use. Typically, this

was because with the current baby boom in the gay community, some donors were booked up by women for months ahead! This is a frustration many women who live in gay-by boom cities like San Francisco currently share:

> The policy of one bank we used was to encourage women to pre-pay for sperm, sometimes for up to six months ahead of time. This effectively put several highly desirable donors out of circulation. This was a terribly frustrating revelation for me, as I had spent days deliberating over donor choices, only to find my top picks were all unavailable. I had to really change my expectation for what kind of donor I was willing to use. Sometimes during the stress of the moment you are willing to compromise, but when I realized I was using a donor whose ethnicity and family health history were not what I really wanted, I had to step back and rethink my decision. Soon afterward, I changed sperm banks entirely and got my top donor pick. Three months later, I was pregnant.—Arlene

ARE YOUR DONORS WILLING TO BE KNOWN?
IF SO, WHEN THE CHILD IS HOW OLD?

There are certainly many more donor choices available to you if you don't ever want to know your donor's identity. That is because it is a relatively a new idea to let children eventually meet their donor fathers. Typically, many donors have been college students just looking to make a little extra money and then walk away. As more and more women use sperm banks, however, the common wisdom of using only unknown donors has changed. Many more mothers would like their children to one day have the option of meeting their donor. There are still few men willing to consider the possibility that one day grown-up offspring may come knocking on their door. More and more, however, women are choosing donors who are willing to be known, sometimes called "yes" donors, if only to give their children the option of finding the men who have contributed to their existence. The average age at which a child can meet a donor father seems to be eighteen, but some banks are allowing younger children to do so.

As a personal note, I'd like to add that in our haste to create families, I feel many lesbians are willing to deny their children the opportunity to seek their biological roots. Knowing many adoptees who as adults were almost frantic to find their biological parents has taught me the wisdom of not imposing our own limitations on our children. The fact that we create these children and want them to grow up in a lesbian family will not alleviate their own eventual quest to know their origins, whether or not we approve. If we use donors who are willing to be known, our children can grow up secure in the knowledge that should they seek to find their donor father, they will be able to do so one day.

Here is an example of an unknown donor's information. As you can see, what you will know about half of your child's genetic makeup is quite small:

Donor # 2213
Race/Ethnicity: Caucasian/German/English
Hair Color/Texture: Light Brown/Wavy
Eye Color: Blue
Skin Tone: Fair
Blood Type: A+
Height: 6'1"
Weight: 185 lbs
Occupation: Fireman
Interests: Nature, Swimming, Film
Religion: Catholic

For known donors, you may find the initial information listed will be about the same, but then once you narrow down your choices, the bank will provide a more detailed family health history for you. Often this will also contain several pages of information, which may include the donor's favorite foods and colors, as well as his reasons for becoming a donor. If you can read these forms at the clinic, there is generally no fee, but if you want a photocopy most banks charge up to $20 each for a printout of only several pages. Just another way to bring in the bucks, I guess!

Questions to Ask About Particular Donors

WHAT IS HIS FAMILY MEDICAL HISTORY?
Make sure you really study the more detailed donor profile. Look for diseases like cancer and heart problems, chronic conditions like eczema and allergies, and genetic problems like dwarfism and color-blindness.

WHAT IS HIS POST-THAW MOTILE SPERM COUNT?
Not all banks will tell you this, and I have yet to ever see it on a donor profile. But if you can find out, it's a good bit of information to know. Multiple sperm work together to penetrate the egg, even though only one will get in and join with that egg. So the more of them that can get to the egg, the better your chances to conceive. Most guys average about 30 to 80 million sperm per cc, but my donor had 210 million per cc. Rather extraordinary, and one of the reasons I chose him!

HAS HE PRODUCED OTHER LIVE CHILDREN? HOW MANY?
Some banks will tell you this only if you ask, and others won't provide the information at all. But if you know a guy's been an active donor for more than a year and no one's ever gotten pregnant by him, I'd pick another guy. My own informal research on this particular issue shows that men with high sperm counts produce more children, and that women get pregnant faster when they use these donors.

WILL THE DONOR BE AVAILABLE IF I WANT MORE CHILDREN?
Most banks will stop using a donor once a set number of women (usually between four and ten) become pregnant by him. Generally, though, they will guarantee repeated use if you want to birth a sibling, but you should always check to make sure...even if at the time you're not sure you'll ever want another child.

What You Should Expect from Your Sperm Bank

COURTEOUS, KNOWLEDGEABLE SERVICE.
Staff should be friendly, empathetic, and willing to answer your questions. Especially when you are first starting out, it's important to have the feeling that clinic staff are on your side. It can be painful and disorienting if you are given wrong information or made to feel as though your concerns are not valid:

> We asked one clinic worker if there was any way to better our chances of having a girl over a boy. We were mostly just curious, but instead of just giving us the information we wanted, she went off on a ten-minute rant about how wonderful her boy children were. We felt belittled and humiliated, and never used their services again.—Barbara

FREQUENT UPDATES OF DONOR LISTS.
If these lists are not updated every six months or so, they will likely include donors who are no longer available.

HOURS OF OPERATION THAT ARE CONVENIENT TO YOU.
If your bank or fertility clinic is only open Monday–Friday 9–5 (and many are), it may not be convenient for you. If you ovulate on a Saturday and can't get an appointment or sperm, you're outta luck that month! Some fertility doctors have actually put women on drugs to regulate their cycles for no other reason than the convenience to their own schedules. It might be time to seek another option at that point.

OPENNESS TO CRITICISM.
If you have a complaint about the way a bank is doing business with you, you should be able to let them know. If someone gave you incorrect information or was rude, you should feel comfortable addressing this. Often, if there is a real problem, you may get a free month of sperm or some other compensation. I'm not talking about suing or other nasty things here. Rather, just as in any other consumer exchange, you should feel empowered to express dissatisfaction and not be intimidated by the "experts." That's all.

Basically, the better informed you are as a client, the easier time you will have using whatever service you choose. Figure on it taking a few months to get into the swing of whichever method you choose to use. It can be an expensive education if things go wrong, but it's almost inevitable that things will once in a while. It's part of this whole mysterious process you're embarking on…part timing, part science, and part magic. And there's just no accounting for magic!

How to Choose a Donor

It used to be that women had few choices about donor selection. Basically, they took what was available through a doctor. Donors were generally medical students affiliated with the clinic. Single women and lesbians were not even allowed to inseminate!

These days, not only are lesbians a large percentage of some sperm banks' business, but you are likely to have a potentially overwhelming number of men to choose from. When you pick a sperm bank, you are basically trusting them to provide you with a mixture of different types of guys. A few of these will be desirable to you, and if all goes well, you will get pregnant by one of them.

Ultimately, the only expert you can count on in this process is yourself. The better educated you are, the more likely you are to feel that you, the paying customer and hopeful parent, are in control of this process.

Selecting a donor is not a decision to take lightly. So the first question you need to ask yourself is, What are you looking for in your future child's genetic makeup? Some things may be obvious to you. For example, you may decide you only want a Caucasian donor, or an African American one. This will narrow the field considerably. But what if you want a biracial child? Or if you're of an unusual biracial mixture yourself and want to duplicate that? If you have a partner, would you prefer that the donor's physical appearance match hers more closely than yours? Do you want someone who has a lot of education? Who has traveled extensively? Who has lots of siblings? And what if you like everything about a donor, till you find out there's a history of breast cancer or eczema in his family? Do you still pick him? Or choose a different guy altogether?

Some donor profiles will seem to just jump out of the page at you (hey, he's got red hair and plays the piano!), but it's also possible you might have to really hunt for one that looks good to you. I would advise taking your time to narrow down your selections to the top five, and not pin all your hopes on just one donor. That one may not be available, or his supply might run out, and you will feel very let down. Also, you might try for a while with one donor and not get pregnant. Sometimes, it will feel empowering to switch, to give yourself a fresh start. Some women have told me they've had a strong adverse reaction after using a certain donor. I would definitely listen to your intuition, and make adjustments accordingly.

> *If you are using an unknown donor, don't be afraid to switch donors if one is not working out for you. We changed three times until we finally got a keeper.—Joani*

The Money Factor

Sperm Bank Costs

Here is an average price list from a typical sperm bank and an explanation of the most common terms you will encounter:

REGISTRATION: $150.
This is a one-time fee some banks charge you for an intake. Not all sperm banks do this, but if it is required, you have to pay it. At this time, a staff member may go over some information like how to chart your cycles and when they are open for pickups of sperm.

HEALTH TESTS: $0–$600.
Most sperm banks require that you be healthy and able to prove it. Many will ask for a minimum of blood tests (proof of HIV status, etc.), but others want many more, such as tests for HTLV-1, CMV, syphilis, rubella, toxoplasmosis, Tay-Sachs, sickle-cell disease, and myco-ureaplasma. These can become expensive. If you have them at the clinic, you will be charged. If you have a regular doctor or are covered by a health plan, you will probably prefer to get them done yourself and just bring in the results.

FROZEN SEMEN: $150 FOR 1 CC.
A cc is a tiny amount of semen in a little plastic vial, which is how sperm comes from the bank. Initially, you may not believe that such a small amount of semen can ever get you pregnant. But each vial should contain millions and millions of sperm, more than enough to get the job done.

INTRAUTERINE: $150–$250.
I really believe that an intrauterine (IUI) is the optimal procedure for achieving pregnancy when you only have one shot a month to try. While there are no hard-and-fast statistics, it seems that by regularly trying IUIs, you will probably cut the time you spend getting pregnant in half. Why? For one thing, you will know the sperm is viable. There's no opportunity for your dry ice to run out, or for the syringe to slip, or for any of the other mishaps that can happen at home. Often, you can even look under a microscope at the clinic after the procedure and see an "extra" drop or two of sperm swimming with life. I was never convinced that the samples we brought home with us were actually capable of making me pregnant. Seeing the semen from my donor so healthy and mobile gave me an emotional boost and really made me believe I would soon get pregnant.

When you have an IUI, the sperm is generally "spun" to remove the active swimmers from the rest of the liquid semen. This concentrated solution is then fed through a tube directly through your cervix and into your uterus. Therefore, the sperm not only is more concentrated but also doesn't have to swim through your mucus, which can be like an obstacle course for the little swimmers. The procedure cuts the sperm's long journey into your body by about five hours by bypassing the trek through your vagina. It's a head start for the sperm and places them a lot closer to the egg. It's a more expensive procedure, but it may prove a lot cheaper in the end than endless rounds of home inseminations. In the end, it may also then prove to be less stressful.

Do IUI's hurt? While there is a chance for some cramping, most women experience no discomfort at all. I felt a slight sensation when the tiny tube was fed through my cervix, and that was about it. It was a lot less messy than an insemination at home, and just as fast.

Some midwives are now skilled in doing intrauterine inseminations for their clients at home. If you are thinking about using a midwife for your birth, you may want to ask her if she is qualified to also help you inseminate. That way you can combine the comfort and intimacy of being in your own home with the greater effectiveness of the IUI method.

Getting pregnant with frozen sperm will cost an average of $300–$600 a cycle if you are inseminating at home, $400–$1000 a cycle if you are using the services of a clinic or bank for procedures such as IUIs.

INTRACERVICAL:
$100 AND UP.

An intracervical is like an intrauterine, except the sperm doesn't quite get as far in as your uterus. It will be placed just on the other side of your cervical opening, or right at the opening. Sometimes it is done because your cervix is partially closed, and the tube used in an intrauterine just won't go farther into your uterus. Despite the fact that an intracervical is potentially less effective than an intrauterine, this is the procedure that finally got me pregnant.

It All Adds Up

Yes, trying to get pregnant can get very expensive! Besides the costs just listed, you may also be spending money on costly fertility drugs. And sometimes there are extra fees for weeknight, weekend, or Sunday hours at clinics, which you may end up paying if your cycle and schedule demand that you inseminate at those times. You may also need to have sperm shipped and/or stored if you do not live near a clinic, or the clinic of your choice. So then you must factor in the cost of renting and/or shipping a liquid nitrogen tank from the bank to store the sperm to keep it cold enough. You will also have to pay to ship it back to the bank. Women who bring sperm home from a bank must buy a cooler to store it in, as well as dry ice each month to keep it cold. And since dry ice loses at least half its volume each day, count on buying lots of ice! Often, there are also extra expenses, such as syringes, temperature charts, and of course, your ovulation predictor kits.

It's true, you may be one of the lucky gals who gets pregnant the first time. However, you should plan on it costing about $500–$1,000 for your first cycle, including lab work and an intake, and about $300–$700 each cycle thereafter. Trying twice a cycle may double your chances, but it will also probably double your costs. The high expense of getting pregnant can add tremendously to the stress of trying to get pregnant. When your finances start to dwindle, take a month or two off to recoup.

Insurance

Some women are lucky enough to have their fertility services covered by their health insurance in full. Others can claim partial coverage. Most women aren't able to claim much. But every policy is different. Ask in advance, so you know what's up, and you may be able to upgrade or change coverage completely to get a break. To avoid being denied coverage, you may need to claim that you have been previously unable to conceive, rather than saying you are a lesbian. Some insurance packages will cover the services of a fertility clinic but not the sperm. Or you may just feel more comfortable using the services of a sperm bank of your choice that costs money, even if you have insurance through a provider like an HMO. Of course, if you don't have insurance, you will end up paying for everything anyway. Some women have said that paying out all this money provided them a financial reality check—if you can't afford to get pregnant, how will you ever afford the costs of a child?

When using the services of a fertility OB/GYN, you might be asked to attend one or more counseling sessions. This is considered a routine procedure for both straight and gay couples, particularly if you are using the services of a sperm bank. However, if you can show that you have already thought through many of the issues involved, you may be able to have these sessions waived.

Most insurance companies don't cover "infertility treatment," which is what artificial insemination is classified as, but most do cover the rest of your maternity expenses— i.e., prenatal exams, hospital or birthing center delivery, etc. Just get the best deal you can. Remember to check out your insurance company's preapproval clauses. I was moments from delivery and on the phone with the damned insurance people—they called the hospital when the first paperwork reached them, and wondered what the heck was happening! Arghhhh! What did they think all those prenatal expenses were for, fun? Dealing with them between contractions was not enjoyable!—Marissa

Trying at Home

What You Will Need for Each Insemination

- A small, six-pack sized cooler to keep the container of sperm in.
- An adequate supply of dry ice to keep the sperm cold.
- A speculum to isolate your cervix.
- A flashlight to see your cervix.
- A needle-less syringe to inseminate.
- A towel to place under your buttocks to absorb spillage of semen.
- Disposable latex gloves for the inseminator to use.

Syringes

It may be difficult to find a place where you can purchase the thin needle-less syringes that are best used for insemination. If you are using a sperm bank and plan to inseminate at home, 10cc syringes will usually be supplied by the bank, but in researching this book I couldn't find any sperm banks which sold the syringes separately. While some drugstore and/or medical supply companies do stock them, you usually need a doctor's prescription to purchase syringes. However, most national drug store chains sell something called a medicine applicator for under $3, used orally to give medicine to children. A medicine applicator is essentially a thick, needle-less syringe and will do the job quite nicely. Some pharmacies even give them out for free! It is ironic that a forbidden syringe can be repackaged as an "oral syringe" (the Walgreen's kit even comes with cleaning brush to scrub it out) and be sold next to diapers and baby bottles in the drugstore! If only they knew!

Our sperm bank was in California, so we pretty much had to guess when we'd be ovulating and needing the sperm shipped. If we were early by more than forty-eight hours, we had to keep the sperm on dry ice, and we had a hard time finding that in the town where we lived. At first we didn't tell Baskin Robbins why we needed the dry ice we'd ask for every month. But after several months of this, they knew what we were doing and were cheering us on.—Angela

When we had our sperm delivered, were we ever surprised to see a cute baby butch lesbian driver handing over the goods. She looked knowingly at the box marked "medical supplies," smiled, said "good luck," and drove off!—Beverly

Many women, particularly women in couples, will prefer to initially try at home to become pregnant. If you are using sperm from a sperm bank, you will have to thaw it according to the clinic's instructions. The most common procedure is to set the frozen sperm vial in warm (not hot) water for about five minutes until it thaws to room temperature and a runny consistency. Note that if the sperm has thawed by accident or has been sitting around outside the cooler for longer than an hour or two, it may not be good. You cannot refreeze it yourself or keep fresh sperm at home in a regular freezer, as keeping sperm frozen requires a *much* colder temperature than that of your refrigerator freezer. Remember also to keep the cooler tightly closed, out of the sun, and wrapped in a towel to help preserve its coldness. You may want to rent a liquid nitrogen tank to avoid losing your sperm if your cooler's dry ice evaporates too quickly.

For the actual insemination, the preferred method these days is to use a needle-less syringe to draw the sperm up. The stereotypical turkey baster will probably not work with the tiny amounts of sperm you buy from a bank. Some women just lie back and squirt the goods in, and let nature take its course. However, if you want to maximize your at-home chances, a speculum (plastic is much nicer than metal) should be used on the woman being inseminated. This enables the person inseminating her to see her cervix, which is the general area to aim for. If you've opened the speculum and can't see the cervix, you will need to adjust the speculum until you do. The cervix, which you will probably need a flashlight to really see, should ideally appear open and a bit wet with clearish mucus. Some women's cervixes may even produce so much mucus when they're fertile that it will be oozing out. This is a good sign of fertility, so don't worry about it blocking the entranceway into your body—the sperm will swim right through it! If you are the person doing the inseminating, be careful not to get overly excited and drop or depress the syringe; the last thing you want to do is shoot the sperm across the room. This actually happened to friends of mine! It may be a good idea to have another friend there to help by holding the flashlight. If you are using a speculum, you'll want to ensure that at least some of the semen is coated on or around the cervix, although you don't want to aim inside the cervix— that can cause infection. The syringe should be depressed slowly and steadily, and withdrawn the same way. Some spillage out of your vagina is inevitable, so don't panic if you feel semen running out of your body. You haven't lost it all, just some extra liquid. Don't worry—it will take your first try or two to get comfortable with the procedure!

Speculums

Check women's health centers, local midwives, or Planned Parenthood for speculums. Plastic reusable speculums can also be mail-ordered from Awakenings Birth Services in San Francisco. See the Resource section for details.

The most embarrassing moment of my pregnancy was when an old girlfriend of my partner's came over and showed us how to place the semen inside me. Of course, I had to "assume the position" for her, and I had never even met her before!—Nadine

Sex after insemination was wonderful! As an incest survivor I felt this was a way of putting men in their proper place. They served a purpose in the creation of a baby without having to be directly involved. Very freeing for me!—Estela

Many women like to elevate their bottoms on pillows or up on the wall for about twenty minutes afterward to allow the sperm a better shot at swimming up into the uterus. This is probably a good idea, although I've heard stories about women inseminating themselves in their car and then driving off to a meeting, and still ending up pregnant. Go figure.

There is certainly an intimacy about trying at home that cannot be duplicated at even the most well-meaning clinic. Especially if you are part of a couple, it will make the nonbiological partner feel much more involved if she's actually the one doing the insemination. It may also be nice to try to incorporate lovemaking into the ritual, although I found I was usually too tense to have sex after or before insemination. Just remember not to use lube. And since some midwives are now doing intrauterine inseminations, at-home IUIs may soon become the preferred method of trying to conceive.

I know of women who plan elaborate conception ceremonies for their at-home tries. These may include a blessing, candles, and poetry. If you take more than a few cycles to conceive, however, you may find that you bother less with these things and get down to business more quickly.

It's a personal choice and won't affect whether you get pregnant. Probably the most important thing you can do for yourself, however, is to *relax* as much as possible.

> *We have a seven-month-old girl conceived on the third try. On that attempt we dimmed the lights and brought out special items from our two other children. We spent thirty minutes in the doctor's office, with my partner lying upside down on the table with her hips raised and me giving her those items one by one.—Terese*

Trying at home can be romantic at first, but using the services of a professional clinic can be more effective in the long term.

> *We did all the right things the first time around and made that try special...and we didn't get pregnant. By try six we were watching Jeopardy! while inseminating. And try fourteen was all-around irritating, with bad scheduling and a hectic day and rotten traffic, and we were sure we had the timing all wrong—and that's when we got pregnant. It was about as romantic as a root canal.—Rebecca*

In my own case, after three or four months of trying, I bacame convinced that there was no way I was ever going to become pregnant at home with frozen sperm. There were just too many variables, such as whether we had thawed the sperm properly, or whether our dwindling supply of dry ice had kept the sperm viable. It was actually a relief to begin going in for my monthly intrauterines at the clinic, because the onus shifted from myself and my lover to them. At Rainbow Flag's clinic we were even able to view some of the sperm sample under the microscope afterward, and watch the few last little sperm swim crazily around on a slide. It was a relief to know that not only had the goods thawed properly, but they were at that very moment dashing merrily along inside me in search of that ever-elusive egg.

Other Options

Using an Anonymous Donor with Fresh Sperm, Through a Middleman

Although using an anonymous donor through a middleman was the way many lesbians got pregnant in the pre-AIDS era, this has pretty much fallen by the wayside now. Health considerations dictate that this method is not safe, as you know nothing about the donor or his health. Legally, it is also not sound, since it is relatively easy for the donor to find out whom he has impregnated.

Sex with a Man

More lesbians and bisexual women than you'd think try to get pregnant by having sex with a man, or at least think about it. There's something so tempting about the thought of joining two warm bodies together in the magical act of trying to conceive a child. It can be so much more appealing than lying spread-eagle under bright lights on a clinic table. Sex is also cheap, and if you enjoy sex with men, it can be fun! Of course, many women find this thought utterly unappealing, and the health and legal risks involved in conceiving this way are many. The man may have an STD, and the courts will consider him the legal father of your child if he claims paternity. Conceivably, this could give him equal access to your long-awaited child! Any lawyer or health care practitioner would wince at the thought of any lesbian considering sex with a man—particularly one you don't know well—to get pregnant. But many women do it, end up having perfectly healthy children, and never have to see the father again. Or they may have decided that the man they are sleeping with will be a known father to the child. In this case, see "The Father Factor," earlier in this chapter.

In my own frustration at not getting pregnant quickly with frozen sperm, I occasionally contemplated flying off to some small town somewhere and having sex a few times during my ovulation week. In fact, I was convinced that I would get pregnant immediately this way. If you are single, it may be very tempting to try this, but if you have a lover, she may have a problem with your sleeping with some dude to get knocked up. In the end, I never could bring myself to do this, and now I'm glad I was more safety-conscious about it all.

CHAPTER 4

Surviving the Roller Coaster:

Ten Tips to Keep You Sane

If there's one thing I learned from the roller coaster, it's that there are no guarantees...and that it's really important to find the humor in it all.—Karin

Only women who are intentionally trying to get pregnant (and paying lots of money to do so, besides!) can appreciate the madness of this process. The rest of the world will have no idea what you're going through. Even if you try for a year or two, people won't comprehend the stress you're feeling. Only those who have lived through it are truly aware of the emotional and physical roller-coaster ride that trying to conceive will throw us onto, and of the two-week life cycle that our lives suddenly revolve around. I'm here to tell you that unless you get pregnant right on your first try, you will most likely be plunged into this world of emotional upheaval. There's no easy way to survive this time, and it won't end until you get pregnant, but the good news is that it *will* end. It may be hard to believe that when you are reading this chapter. I myself remember thinking that this roller coaster was now a permanent condition, and I was gonna be riding it forever!

I've always believed in the power of distraction. Go to lots of movies. Go for long, energetic walks. Decide to reorganize your bookshelves or do some early Christmas shopping. Every time you start to talk—or even think—about the baby thing, actively change the subject.—Kia

Plan to not be pregnant, and think about the next try. So either you're all prepared for the disappointment, or you get to be surprised and do happy dances about how there won't be a "next" time. And don't do a pregnancy test too early—you don't want to get a negative result and your period on the same day. A definite downer!—Mary

If I can offer any consolation at all, let me reassure you that once you conceive, you'll look back on this time and say, "Oh, I guess it wasn't so bad." That may seem unbelievable now, but when you're fighting off morning sickness or feeling that baby move around in your belly, the awful months of trying will have slipped almost completely out of your head. And when your baby is born, you might just decide you love the first so much that a second would be a good idea. Yes, you might one day willingly submit to this process all over again!

But for now...some tips on how to take care of yourself, and your relationship, so that you can survive this most stressful of times.

1. Take Care of Yourself First

Self-care is absolutely the most important part of this whole process. This is a time of unbelievable stress for most of us, and there won't be many people around who understand how trying it all is. Therefore, do everything you can to be gentle with yourself now. Get enough sleep, eat well, indulge in a monthly massage, take long baths, and commune with whatever Goddess you believe in. Don't give in to drinking too much or other unhealthy ways of dealing with stress. Once you can relax as much as possible about this process, it will become easier to bear it and be able to keep trying. At the same time, be gentle with your lover if you have one, especially if you are doing this together. Trying to get pregnant is a hard thing for couples, and many break up during this time. Don't let wanting a baby destroy your partnership.

If you are doing this as a couple, it is essential to have a rock-solid relationship. Our relationship always came first and was never compromised by our attempts to get pregnant.—Margie

2. Understand That It's Probably Going to Take a While

Sure, some people get lucky the first time, and we all hope that it's going to be us. I have friends who have conceived on their first try and are convinced it should be that easy for everyone. Others have the humility to know that they were just lucky. But for the rest of us, surviving this really difficult time becomes a bit easier if we can understand that especially with frozen sperm, conception usually takes at least a few tries. That's why I always recommend trying at home a time or two just for the experience, then stepping up the effectiveness of your methods, perhaps with an intrauterine at the clinic.

> My girlfriend and I are using the IUI method with the help of an infertility doctor and Clomid. When we first started planning to have a baby, we never thought it would be this much work. No one told us about the time involved looking through donor catalogs, trying to find that "perfect donor" and then living through those long two-week intervals that our lives seemed to be spent in. We got through it by thinking of how worth it it would all be in the end.—Sarah

Additionally, you may want to wait a few months before you announce to everyone that you're trying...otherwise, you'll get asked every month by well-wishers if it's worked. Unless people have been through this themselves, they won't know that instead of appearing supportive, they just come across as irritating.

> If you don't want everyone asking you every month if you are finally pregnant, limit the people who know you're trying. We told many people, and every month it was very painful each time we'd get asked again if it happened yet.—Caroline

3. Realize That Your Life Will Now Be Divided into Two-Week Cycles

> The anxiety of not knowing if I'm pregnant is unbelievable. I never imagined it would be like this. The two-week waiting period is driving us nuts!—Leila

Sure, weeks used to flow by without much notice, but that's all changed now. Once you start trying to conceive a baby, every month of your life will go something like this:

STAGE 1: You'll get your period and cry for a day. You'll bleed for a few days, then call the sperm bank (or your donor) and let them know you will need their services this month. You will start taking your temperature and watching for signs of fertile mucus. You will become more agitated and excited each day. You'll pee on a few ovulation sticks and watch them turn blue, or not. When all signs are a go that you're on the brink of popping out your egg, you'll make an appointment with the sperm bank or donor. Insemination will happen, either in your home, trying to be romantic, or spread-eagle on the clinic table under bright lights. You will tremble with excitement at the prospect that this could be the time, even while you are marveling at the inhumanity of the whole damn process.

STAGE 2: Now that you are inseminated, you will anxiously take your temperature every day to see if it falls. You will become a hypochondriac examining every sign of possible early pregnancy or PMS. Your girlfriend will come to loathe the thermometer beeping first thing in the morning. She will tell you to calm down when you exclaim excitedly that your temperature is still high. You will drive your friends crazy asking, "Do you think I could be pregnant this time?" You will stop drinking alcohol and going hot-tubbing "just in case." You will be sure you are pregnant. Then you will bleed, you will cry, and the nightmare will begin again.

4. Keep Believing It Could Happen Any Time

After eight years together, my partner and I decided to have a baby. We decided to try for a year, but after eleven months of taking my temperature, checking those lovely cervical fluids, arguing over whether the blue line on the ovulation test stick was "blue enough," we were still not pregnant. It is such a trying road when month after month you obsess about something so important.

Before we went in for our twelfth and last insemination I learned some devastating family news and decided I wouldn't try that time. My partner encouraged me to go, knowing I would regret it later if I didn't. Two weeks later we were shopping, buying a box of tampons and a pregnancy test, knowing we'd need one of them the next day. And now I sit holding my four-month-old son, the most incredibly gorgeous baby to ever grace this planet. I guess my message is to never give up. Keep the faith; you never know what miracles await you.—Wendy

That story pretty much says it all. I can't absolutely guarantee that you'll conceive any more than I can predict a major earthquake, but I can tell you that Wendy's story is typical. The time I conceived I was convinced that it couldn't possibly happen that month. I have a beautiful baby girl now just to prove how very wrong I was.

It's really important to know that if you don't get pregnant the first time and have to try again, it's not because you didn't do all the right things at the right time. Don't blame yourselves! Don't waste a moment's stress thinking, "If only we'd done X first" or "If only we'd done Y second" or "If only we'd stood on our heads every second Tuesday." You have to step back and let nature take its course, which is a good first lesson in parenting: you are not 100 percent in control anymore!—Ruth

5. Find Support Wherever You Can

I live in San Francisco and am a pretty well-connected person, but I still felt as though I were inventing the wheel every menstrual cycle. The fact is, even with the so-called gay-by boom in full effect, trying to conceive is a tremendously isolating experience. You will probably feel like you are the only dyke in the world who has ever gone through this. As much as they may be supportive in the beginning, your friends will soon get bored with your monthly angst, so look elsewhere. Places to start are friends of friends who are trying (call them, even if they're strangers, because they may soon be your best friends), online bulletin boards (the lesbian parenting board on America Online kept me sane during this process), and support groups—even if you have to start your own. In some cities there may be "insemination support groups" specifically for lesbians, possibly offered through the practices of lesbian midwives. Even just finding the one sympathetic person at the sperm bank will make the whole process much more humanizing. You will also find yourself bonding with straight women in ways you wouldn't have previously imagined. In fact, your mostly childless dyke friends will have no frame of reference for your entire, all-consuming pregnancy experience, and they may be unsympathetic throughout. Straight women, however, many of whom have had children or are trying to, will immediately relate to your struggle, if they are at all enlightened. Sexual boundaries may melt before your eyes. During my whole pregnancy, one or two dyke friends, my online chat board, and a whole bevy of straight customers at my book shop who gave me the most backup. Get support wherever you can, and don't be afraid to reach out for it from unlikely sources.

6. Don't Hang Out with Nonsupportive People

It's isolating enough having to educate everyone you care about, so don't waste energy on the cads. I had to learn this the hard way, when I went out to dinner with dyke friends of my girlfriend, during my first trimester. Given how sick I was feeling the first few months, it was all I could do that night to drag myself out to the restaurant to meet these new gals. Somehow, during their line of very invasive questioning about the whole ordeal, my girlfriend let slip that my sex drive was way down. No big surprise, given that I felt like puking for sixteen weeks straight! Thereby one of those gals let launch a huge explanation of why she thought I had this problem, none of which was supportive or well informed. I was humiliated beyond belief. There is no room for this in your pregnancy. You will be emotionally volatile enough without acquaintances merrily spewing forth their uninformed ideas. Pitch people like this right out of your life! Others to avoid are people who think parenthood is for the birds, people who hate children, people who have a disturbing analysis of why you aren't getting pregnant, and anyone who thinks queers shouldn't have kids.

7. Expect Your Body to Freak Out, But Try Not to Obsess So Much That You Really Flip

Yes, expect all sorts of disconcerting things to happen to you from the stress of trying to get pregnant. For me, it meant that my usually regular twenty-eight-to-thirty-day menstrual cycle started jumping anywhere from twenty-six to thirty-four days. Some months I'd have fertile mucus, others I wouldn't. I got a weird infection in my mouth. I broke out more. I thought (and my girlfriend did, too) that I was going insane. Relax; it's (unfortunately) normal.

> *Prepare yourself to become obsessive. You'll be drinking cough syrup, brewing up horrible-tasting teas, and doing your ovulation tests in the office restroom.*—Zada

8. Take Time Out When You Need It

If you find that you are literally on the edge of a nervous breakdown, take time out. Skip a month or two to regain your sanity, your finances, or both. It is extremely hard to stop in the middle of this process and take a breather. You will feel the clock ticking and wonder each time you miss a month, "Could this have been the time?" Yet, your body and brain need a rest from the tremendous strain of the whole process. Maybe you could justify it by skipping the astrological signs you don't want your kid to be, or come up with some other equally strange—but valid—reason. Some studies have shown that those who actively engage in stress reduction, meditation, and visualization became pregnant sooner. Even if you don't believe that, it's still important to keep your body and mind in the best shape you can during this process, and I'm convinced that if you're too stressed out, you won't conceive. Once I finally chilled out, I got pregnant.

9. Start Indulging in Parenting Books and Magazines

Parenting books and magazines will make you feel connected to the world of parenting, even if just peripherally. Go to your nearest independent bookstore and peruse the racks, or subscribe to magazines like

Alternative Family, a gay-oriented parenting mag (see Resources for contact info), and *Parenting Magazine*, a mainstream but gay-friendly glossy. If you start reading these publications now you'll be all the more informed later about things like potty training and ear infections. And all the pictures of cute kids in the mags will no doubt cheer you up as you wonder what your own little tyke will look like. Especially if you're feeling that parenthood is all just a shaky dream, display these books and magazines on your coffee table, so you'll know, and everyone else will too, that you're serious about this endeavor.

10. Reevaluate Your Process as Necessary

The conception roller coaster has many twists and turns along the way, so don't be rigid about anything. Things I changed my mind about over the course of the year it took me to get pregnant: To sleep with a guy or use frozen sperm? To use a known or unknown donor? Which specific donor to use? To change donors after a few unsuccessful tries? To inseminate at home or at the clinic? To move from simple inseminations to more invasive (but more effective) intrauterines? To inseminate once a cycle or twice? Or more? To change sperm banks altogether? To take fertility drugs or not? Which ones? For how long? Most women go through a whole litany of decision making as they wind their way toward becoming pregnant. The little line in the sand you're not willing to go beyond will change with time. Allow it to.

Final Survival Tip:

Punch anyone who asks you every month, "So, are you pregnant yet?"
    Just kidding...sort of!

CHAPTER 5

What if You Can't Get Pregnant?

On the path to pregnancy, there are often many detours. One of the hardest to deal with is the growing realization that because you don't seem to be getting pregnant, something might be wrong.

Everyone who tries to get pregnant hopes that conception will happen quickly, but we all know realistically that it can take a while. That may be especially true for women who are over thirty-five or using frozen sperm. You know by now that riding the conception roller coaster is a normal experience. So you may not question just *why* you can't seem to get pregnant when everyone you know is pushing around a baby carriage. Even if you wanted to consult with someone sooner, many infertility doctors won't even see you unless you've tried for a year.

> *We've found that most doctors don't want to do invasive procedures unless there is a good reason to suspect there is a problem. I would talk to your doctor about getting some testing done earlier on rather than waiting a year. Make sure he or she understands the expense and emotional trauma you are going through every month. I work with physicians and think many will modify their usual year's wait if you make a strong case.—Lynda*

If you're trying to conceive at home with the help of a sperm bank, you might not even know about the possibility of fertility drugs. Most banks will not mention them until you bring it up. I think they're used to it taking a while for women to conceive with their services, and of course their profits depend on women continuing to use their product. So aside from requiring basic health tests, they may not push for more intervention.

All women who have problems conceiving should consult a fertility specialist called a reproductive endocrinologist, and not rely on their regular OB/GYN. — Leland Traiman, director, Rainbow Flag Health Services and Sperm Bank

The Next Step

However, once eight months to a year have passed, the frustration level for many women is past the boiling point. You will be asking yourself every day what could possibly be wrong. Why aren't you getting pregnant? What can you do about it?

The best first step is to get a thorough checkup, if you haven't done so already. The next is to ask your regular OB/GYN to recommend a reproductive endocrinologist, or RE. These are specialists who are used to seeing women with fertility problems and know what to look for, what tests to do, and what treatments you may need. They will be much more aggressive than regular doctors about offering up-to-date suggestions for tests and procedures.

What Could Be Wrong?

There are many medical problems that can interfere with a woman's ability to conceive and carry a healthy baby to term. These include fibroids, endometriosis, or a blocked fallopian tube. Endometriosis can in particular be a stumbling block to pregnancy. It's a disease that often causes pain but may go unnoticed until fertility questions come up. The condition occurs when some of the tissue that normally lines the uterus grows elsewhere in the body, particularly around or on the ovaries.

> I have endometriosis and have been trying to get pregnant for a while. Information regarding endo and pregnancy is very confusing. Every doctor I saw gave me a different answer for everything. And my nurse practitioner told me I will never get pregnant with endo (even with it removed) unless I do in vitro. But I called an infertility clinic and they said they see women with endo get pregnant all the time. I think you really have to be willing to read a lot of material on your own, ask a lot of questions, and be an advocate for yourself.—Beverly

You may even want to make sure that you are actually ovulating, something that charting your temperature can help determine.

> I was charting my temperatures and noticed that they never went up, which they should if you are ovulating. I called the doctor and she told me to come in for a progesterone test. Turns out my progesterone was too low and I wasn't ovulating. So I started taking 50mg of Clomid to help me ovulate.—Enid

A good RE will leave no stone unturned on the road to getting you pregnant. Of course, what you can afford will depend on your income and also the type of medical coverage you have. But you should always feel that the doctor is empathetic to your particular medical situation, that you are kept appraised of your treatment options, and that you are dealt with in an open and nondiscriminatory way. If you have any doubts about whether the doctor is being as aggressive as you would like with treatments, or if you feel you (and your partner) are not being treated in a fair manner, it is best to raise the issue or switch doctors.

> I had fertility problems and ended up getting a hysterosalpingogram [an X-ray examination of the uterus and fallopian tubes that may reveal, through the injection of dye, whether there are blockages or other problems], which was a rather unpleasant procedure.

I couldn't see the monitor, I didn't know what was happening, and they wouldn't let my partner into the room. I was told my tubes were blocked and I would need laparoscopic surgery to clear it up. We decided from that point on that we needed to present a united front and would only accept treatment from doctors who treated us respectfully individually and as a couple.—Maureen

If trying to conceive itself is stressful, you can imagine how hard all these added problems can make it feel. Between doctor appointments, treatments, and inseminations, you may truly feel that your attempts to get pregnant are ruling your life.

Medical intervention is expensive and hard to deal with since you have to go to the doctor some seven times over two weeks for ultrasounds, consultations, and inseminations. It's very time-consuming and extremely stressful.—Tara

I found that health insurance for infertility treatments is a big issue for many lesbians. I had insurance that covered my visits with my reproductive endocrinologist and surgery for endometriosis, but nothing else. I had to switch insurers and then found that not even a consultant appointment was covered. I pay for procedures out of pocket and just spent more than $400 in fertility drugs this month.—Jane

Friends may think you are crazy to go through so much in the quest for a child, and it may be hard to relate to anyone who hasn't been through a similar ordeal. Yet, it can also be empowering to feel at last that you know what is wrong, and that you are doing something productive about it. While fertility problems may be that detour I mentioned earlier, they are certainly not the end of the road for many women. Try to find at least one sympathetic, knowledgeable person to share your problems with, even if it means joining a support group for straight women.

Having friends with whom I can share all the woes of infertility has proved vital in keeping my sanity during this process. When I went for my latest insemination a friend of mine who'd also had infertility problems came with me and brought her seven-week-old baby. When I had my IUI, which I found painful, my friend put her little boy in my arms, and I held him while the insemination took place. I figure if he can't bring me good luck, no one can.— Ana

Alternative Treatments for Infertility

I tried for nine months to get pregnant, and my doctor was not very encouraging, since he felt my chances were poor. I finally got pregnant after going to a Chinese herbalist. Don't believe everything a doctor tells you, and by all means seek "alternative" treatment. It may make all the difference.—Caroline

Before you take drugs, there are other options available to increase your fertility. Many women try acupuncture, herbs, and even Chinese teas. You can visit an herbalist, Chinese doctor, or other alternative healers with the specific goal of getting pregnant. You don't have to wait till you receive a pronouncement of infertility to seek out these treatments, either. Many women seek out such treatments concurrent with medical care, for a more holistic approach to conception and pregnancy.

The longer you try to get pregnant, the more desperate you are likely to feel. As time goes by, you may be more willing to take fertility drugs, whereas several months earlier there was no way you would have. We all have a line we're not willing to cross regarding medical intervention. Frequently, this line gets pushed back further and further as time goes by, the periods keep coming, and there's no baby in sight. This is normal, so don't beat yourself up about it. Even though my periods were regular, after six unsuccessful inseminations, I too was considering asking about fertility drugs. Thankfully, attempt number seven turned out to be the lucky one for me.

Fertility Drugs

There are several reasons why some women experience significant problems conceiving a child. One of the most treatable and most common conditions that prevents women from getting pregnant is irregular periods—and therefore irregular ovulation. If women don't ovulate, they are said to be "anovulatory." Causes of this include glandular problems and certain types of hormonal imbalances. It can be really difficult to know when to inseminate (never mind to get pregnant!) when you're not able to pinpoint your ovulation.

By far the most popular way of coping with this is by going on a fertility drug called Clomid (clomiphene citrate). Clomid regulates ovulation by stimulating estrogen production. Clomid has a high rate of success among women without significant fertility problems, and many get pregnant within two or three cycles of using it. The drug is taken orally, with a typical dosage being one or two pills of 50 mg per day for five days. The average cost of each pill is about $10. If it is going to work, it generally does so in the first month or two of use. Sometimes Clomid is combined with a follicle-ripening drug called Pergonal (human menopausal gonadotropin, hMG). Leland Traiman, director of Rainbow Flag Health Services, calls Pergonal a "quantum leap above" Clomid in effectiveness. Pergonal is expensive, however, and is injected rather than taken orally.

Like any intervention, Clomid is not a miracle drug, and some physicians believe it is over-prescribed. Clomid can dry up helpful cervical mucus (some women are given estrogen to prevent this) and may increase the risk of ovarian cancer later in a woman's life. It also carries about a ten percent chance of leading to multiple births, since it can, according to Traiman, "kick more eggs out of your ovaries."

Some women may have naturally low progesterone levels and cannot support a pregnancy even if sperm meets egg. They are said to have an "inadequate luteal phase," since the luteal phase is the time after ovulation. These women may be prescribed extra progesterone via pills, suppositories, or injection to keep them from menstruating. With the boost of extra progesterone, any fertilized eggs have a chance to implant and not be miscarried. Although it may take some time before a woman suspects she may have this problem, once diagnosed with a blood test, she's often successfully treated.

There are other even stronger drugs available, often in conjunction with high-tech procedures such as in vitro fertilization. These drugs are very expensive and can cause serious side effects, but these may not be an obstacle if you are determined to have a baby.

Unfortunately, there are also fertility problems which are impossible to diagnose. Some women just do not get pregnant no matter what they try. Still others may have structural problems of the uterus or cervix, often as the result of exposure to DES in the womb. DES (diethylstilbestrol) was given to women to prevent miscarriage from the 1940s through the early 1970s, and the daughters of women who took it often have a hard time conceiving and carrying a pregnancy to term. If you ascertain you are a "DES daughter" you should consult a specialist before you begin trying to get pregnant.

Remember that some fertility drugs including Pergonal (but usually not Clomid) can affect the results of ovulation predictor kits.

What Some Women Have to Say About Clomid and Other Fertility Drugs

Don't be afraid of fertility drugs. Just because we're lesbians doesn't mean that we have to do everything naturally, and it can waste a lot of time. I waited through nine months of inseminations before wondering whether I ought to ask about fertility drugs. Now looking back at my two pregnancies, I realize there's no way I would have gotten pregnant either time without Clomid. And lookie at what I got for it!—Maria

I had a low progesterone level, which was picked up very early in the process by my fertility specialist. I had to bump up the level of Clomid to 150mg before it raised my progesterone enough to be at a normal level. Two tries at a normal level and we were pregnant.—Katrina

When we started trying to conceive, my partner was on Clomid because of a history of irregular ovulation. After six months of trying at home (frozen sperm, two inseminations per month) we decided we needed some help. We were referred to a reproductive endo–

One last word on fertility drugs. As more and more women use them to become pregnant, the rates of multiple births continue to go up. Because more eggs are produced with fertility drugs, the chances that you'll have to deal with this possibility are very real. It's important before you begin using these drugs that you understand their side effects and consider whether you're prepared to have twins, triplets, or even more children! The issue of selective reduction, whereby certain less viable eggs are discarded once fertilized, is a topic under much discussion. Unfortunately, selective reduction can also lead to miscarriage.

crinologist, who kept my partner on Clomid and added Metrodin (to stimulate egg production) and hCG (to help launch the eggs). The first time we tried this combo we got pregnant! Needless to say, we are very thankful to Western medicine for the help we got in having our twin boys.—Gwyneth

My regular OB/GYN doesn't do inseminations in her office, so we decided to try using a fertility doctor. First thing he did was check my progesterone level, saw that it was too low, and put me on Clomid. I could have tried getting pregnant for a whole year before we realized it wouldn't happen. What a nightmare that would have been! I was pregnant three months later.—Leesa

I took Clomid in combination with Repronex injections. I have heard that women have hugely varied reactions to the drugs, from depression to elation, but I was symptom-free.—Anya

I took 50mg of Clomid for two months and got pregnant on the second try. I went through a fertility specialist and he used an ultrasound to check for viable eggs, then I was inseminated by IUI. The only thing I didn't like about the drug was that it caused me lots of cramping. But it was worth it!—Stephanie

Taking It One Step Further

I tried for a year to get pregnant at home with frozen sperm. Then I had three IUIs, again with no luck. After taking off a few months to chill out, I decided to just throw down all my money and try in vitro fertilization. The first time I tried it, I got pregnant. Drastic, maybe, but I got my baby!—Lois

Some coupled lesbians who have trouble getting pregnant will switch roles, with the second woman attempting pregnancy. And some women will donate an egg to their partner for her to carry, allowing both women to share in the pregnancy experience. These are not options available to straight couples! Of course, there are a few other options for those who are trying to conceive and have the money, time, and willpower to attempt them. Besides increasingly potent injectable drugs, these other methods include in vitro fertilization, gamete intrafallopian transfer (in which a woman's mature eggs are taken from the ovaries and placed with sperm into the fallopian tubes), and even more high-tech marvels. In vitro fertilization, a process in which a woman's eggs are harvested and fertilized outside her body and then replaced in her uterus to mature, is becoming an increasingly popular—though expensive—option. It can run up to $10,000 an attempt, but a very high percentage of women get pregnant the first time or two they try. Still, while some women have luck with these procedures, for others, they are simply another expensive round of frustration and side effects. Most lesbians don't investigate these options, given their high cost and the decreased emphasis many of us place on the importance of carrying on our own genetic line. When we bump up against the bigger walls, we may consider options like adoption instead. But you might want to at least talk to a fertility expert for more information on these types of treatments.

Miscarriage

My first pregnancy ended at about three weeks. I'm sure I noticed only because we knew I was pregnant and were paying such close attention. I had been feeling unwell and then got a period that was heavy, clumpy, and just not normal. I know that feeling as sick as I did, and the pregnancy ending as it did, meant that all was not well, and it was probably for the best that this happened. However, it's been several years and I still wonder and mourn about what might have been. Three months after this loss, I got pregnant again and had a healthy pregnancy and delivery.—Francesca

We had a miscarriage at about ten weeks into our first pregnancy. It is a grieving process like any other. Allow yourselves time to heal and hold each other close. It is such a hard time, but having this experience does at least show you can get pregnant. Keep the faith and ask your doctor if there is anything that you could do next time to increase your success, like progesterone suppositories.—Audre

After a very sad miscarriage, Sally was told she had diabetes. It took us a year and a half and a lot of learning to get her blood sugar under control so we could get pregnant again.—Carla

Statistics show that most women who suffer miscarriage do go on to have a healthy pregnancy. While obviously there can be circumstances that indicate a serious health problem in the mother, often there is nothing really wrong and the miscarriage is no one's fault. Nature has her ways of dealing with imperfect fetuses, and the most common is to flush them out of the mother's body before they become viable. It's estimated that as many as one-third of all pregnancies end in an early miscarriage before the first twenty weeks. A miscarriage may manifest itself as a heavy period, or you may have cramping and clotting. Call a doctor immediately if you suspect anything is wrong or have any bleeding or cramps after a positive pregnancy test. Women who are older than thirty-five may have more miscarriages, but they can happen to women of any age. Because miscarriage can be a sign of maternal disease, including chlamydia, rubella, and lupus, you should always get a checkup after a miscarriage and before attempting pregnancy again.

Coming to the Fork in the Road

Don't forget about all the women who've gone through extreme measures and many years in their journey to pregnancy. I've tried home insemination, IUIs, fresh sperm, frozen sperm, Clomid, Pergonal, in vitro treatments, acupuncture, hypnosis, and a lot of therapy! As lesbians it's difficult enough to find support for what I consider a natural part of being a woman. But I found that the most devastating thing about infertility is the guilt and shame associated with it and the lack of support, particularly in the lesbian community.—Jess

It's a sad fact that not every woman who wants a baby can have one biologically. Many lesbians who have waited till their forties to try to get pregnant may find that their bodies tell them it's too late, either through multiple miscarriages, or simply the lack of a pregnancy.

At some point, we may have to come to a fork in the road along our journey to parenthood. On one side is the road to biological motherhood, but another, equally valid road beckons. It may be heartbreaking initially to give up the biological path. But once you do, a whole other world will open up to you.

You might make peace with the decision not to bear a child, and decide further not to have children in your life at all. But besides biological motherhood, there are many other ways to have children in your life, including mentoring, fostering, coparenting, surrogacy (though the cost of this can run up to $60,000), and adoption. Of course, you can explore all these options even if you're fertile. Unfortunately, depending on where you live, you will find that there may be archaic and homophobic laws barring gay people from adopting or fostering. Usually, however, there are ways around the system. Many women adopt as single people, and foster parent evaluations can be handled in the same way. Of course, no one likes to lie, but sometimes it's necessary. In other cases, it won't even be an issue. Some countries, like China, accept single women as adoptive parents. In fact, lesbians often choose to adopt babies from China. Given that China prefers parents to be over thirty-five years old and have no other children, it's a wonderful parenting option for older women. As you may know, China also has an abundance of girl children needing homes.

Finally, if none of these options pan out, know that there will always be children around you to love. You can volunteer at schools or libraries, become a Big Sister or a camp counselor, or even become a favored auntie to a friend with children. It's certainly not the same as giving birth or having your "own" child. But what a gift you will be able to give to children already around you in your world.

CHAPTER **6**

So You're Finally Pregnant!

Welcome to the World of Eating, Sleeping, and Puking

Is It Pregnancy—Or Just PMS?

If you're like most lesbians trying to get pregnant, immediately after insemination, you will begin thinking you notice signs of pregnancy. This contrasts greatly with the majority of straight women, many of whom might not even get a clue till they miss a period (or two!) and subsequently upchuck in the toilet. Of course, because lesbians have to be so methodical about all this, and it's costing us a fortune besides, we'll be the ones counting the hours till our period is one minute late!

Because most pregnancy books are written for straight women, they usually assume you've already missed a period before they fill you in on a bare minimum of symptoms. But here we can acknowledge the truth: if you've never been a hypochondriac by nature, you will become one when you start trying to conceive. You'll fully believe (and rightly so) that every possible little symptom *may be a sign* of pregnancy. So let's just get a few facts out of the way.

How Do You Know You're Pregnant?

Some women claim to know the minute they inseminate if it has taken. Others want to believe this but are proven wrong when their period blood comes. The truth is probably that when we're hoping we're pregnant, every possible sign becomes greatly magnified. It doesn't help to know that the very early signs of pregnancy are exactly like the symptoms of PMS. In fact, the month I actually got pregnant, I was convinced I couldn't be, because I had such bad PMS-type symptoms. I thought I was going to bleed any minute, and I refused to break down and take a pregnancy test till day 34 of my usually twenty-eight-to-thirty-day cycle.

What to Look For

If you want to hone in on very early signs of pregnancy, here are some things to look for. These can be felt in some women as early as a few days after insemination.

Very Early Pregnancy Signs

- Your breasts start becoming sore.
- You may notice a heightened sense of smell.
- You may begin feeling slightly nauseated or even throw up.
- You may have some slight spotting around the time of your period (from implantation of the egg).
- You may be tired and feel emotionally vulnerable.

Much like PMS, no? So how do you tell the difference? You really can't, unless something obvious happens, like you throw up. And let's hope you have as little of that as possible!

Taking a Pregnancy Test

Most pregnancy tests operate on the same principle. They test for the hormone called hCG (human Chorionic Gonadotrophin) in the urine. So it doesn't matter too much what brand you get or how much you spend. What matters most is that you wait until at least the first day of your missed period to test. When the egg is fertilized, it has a journey of about two weeks in your body till it implants itself in your uterus. Until it implants, the hormone will not register and you will not get a positive result, even if you're actually pregnant. So save that $15 and wait a few days if you can. I know it's hard!

Most tests are easy to use. You simply hold one end of a stick under your morning urine stream, or collect some urine in a clean jar and dip

What's Happening in There?

Weeks 1–2 You aren't even pregnant yet, but these two weeks, the first weeks of your menstrual cycle, count as the first bit of your pregnancy. That's why you'll be forty weeks pregnant—a whopping ten months—before your baby arrives. Now is when the body prepares for the possibility of pregnancy, with the eggs ripening in fluid-filled sacs called follicles.

Week 3 This is the magic week! Ovulation occurs when the ripened egg is swept into the fallopian tube, and if you're to become pregnant, it will be penetrated by the one sperm that's won the race to do so. The egg immediately closes itself to other sperm and begins to divide, floating down the fallopian tube toward the uterus.

Weeks 4–5 This is the time you will probably miss a period and suspect you may be pregnant. Of course, if you are like most lesbians trying to get pregnant, you will have already stocked up on pregnancy tests! The ball of cells, now an embryo, is about a quarter inch long and already has a placenta and umbilical cord.

Weeks 6–8 The embryo has a beating heart but is only about an inch long, about the size of a large bean or berry. It already has small arms and the beginning of toes, ears, and eyelids.

Weeks 9–10 Your baby is now an inch-long fetus that moves, has discernible genitals, and almost looks like a teeny, tiny human being.

Weeks 11–13 Your baby is growing rapidly as you approach the end of your first trimester. It should be close to three inches long now and weigh about half an ounce. It is a fully formed miniature human being that even has fingernails! By week 13 you will most likely be able to hear the whoosh of its heartbeat with the aid of a doppler.

the test stick in. There is a "control" line that is purple or some other color, and then a space for a test result to develop, which should match the control line. If there is no result, you are not pregnant, or you have tested too early, and it's back to the roller coaster again.

If you are pregnant, the stick will display a reading in the test line; even if the result is very faint, you are pregnant. There is no such thing as a little bit pregnant! Some women leave the room and wait a few minutes until the test is done to go in and see the results. Not me! I sat there and watched as that second line came up so fast and so strong that all I could do was sit there and say, "Oh my God, oh my God," over and over. The elation I felt at that moment was overwhelming.

Of course, if you're like me, you won't believe that you actually could get pregnant, so you'll probably go buy at least one more test and try again. But the results will be the same. And sooner or later, you'll have to accept that you really are pregnant. So let me be the first to offer congratulations on what could be one of the most exciting moments in your life. Yes, you're finally pregnant! Congratulations! You really did it! Now prepare to start believing...

You Know...But Should You Tell?

After all your planning and trying and hoping, it may be tempting to want to tell everyone your happy news right away. I know I could barely restrain myself from shouting, "I'm pregnant!" at the top of my lungs as I walked down the street in my neighborhood. Because as lesbians we're actively trying to get pregnant, we tend to find out very early if we're pregnant or not—often we know on the first day of our missed period. But while you may want to tell everyone right away, there are a few reasons to wait. The main one is that most miscarriages happen very early on in a pregnancy, often before most women are even aware they're pregnant.

This type of miscarriage may take the form of a very heavy late period, so if you didn't know you were pregnant, you might not even notice. Women who have shared their pregnancy news early on only to miscarry say that it is a very painful experience. For not only have their hopes for pregnancy been dashed, but they have to tell everyone that they lost the baby. They may also have to deal with constant questions like "So how's the baby?" from people who don't yet know of the loss.

However, often the news is just so exciting, particularly if you've been successful after a long period of trying, that you'll want to tell people, albeit selectively, right from the start. Usually women tell their partner first, then perhaps a select circle of good friends and close family members. Then the news will start spreading, so you may want to actively plan who finds out, and when. Otherwise, there may be some hurt feelings if friends don't hear the word right from you!

How Will People React?

> When I told my mother I was finally pregnant after months of trying, her first reaction was, "Are you sure that's what you want?" I was really hurt, because it seemed like she was saying it was only a mistake! She never asked my straight brother that, and their son was unplanned!—Mimi

> My mother was cautious about my partner and me having a baby. She especially didn't understand how the baby fit into her world, since it was my wife who had him. But once she saw the baby, all misgivings were behind her. You should hear her sweet-talk the baby now! He's the light of her life!—Roberta

The reaction many of us will worry about most is that of our parents. It's true that for some parents, this is the best news that you could ever deliver, and they'll share your joy right from moment one. If you don't have living parents, it may be sad not to be able to share news of an upcoming grandchild with them. If you're estranged from your family, as some gay people are, you may decide to wait to tell them or hope the news will bring you closer. And the fact is, it probably will. Even if they don't like your "lifestyle" or your partner, or don't approve of your being a single parent, once they see their grandchild, they'll probably be in love. It may be hard for some parents to initially accept a grandchild as theirs if it is a child your partner, not you, has borne. But time has a way of healing, and if they see that you are a dedicated parent to the child, and very much a part of a family unit, eventually they'll probably come around.

Obviously, telling supportive friends your good news will be the easy part. But how will more casual acquaintances react? Many lesbians do not understand why some dykes want to become mothers. They may give you a hard time about it, or ask offensive or invasive questions about your methods of conceiving, your pregnancy, or your ability to parent a child. Remember, you do not have to answer any question that makes you uncomfortable or defend your right to have a child, to anyone—even other lesbians! With work colleagues and other straight folks out there in the general population, you may experience more curiosity than overt homophobia, depending on where you live. It's still true that some people can't hide the fact that they believe bringing children up in a gay household is distasteful. However, you need to remember that you will be setting the example here. Showing your happiness and that you're prepared to be a good mother will go further than any argument about the appropriateness of your family. And as more and more lesbians have children, and lesbian families appear to be truly everywhere, prejudice will be chipped away.

Dec 2002 ⌐
Jan 2003 ⌐

Your Due Date

January	1	2	3	4	5	6	7	8	9	10	11	12	13	14	15	16	17	18	19	20	21	22	23	24	25	26	27	28	29	30	31
Oct. / Nov.	8	9	10	11	12	13	14	15	16	17	18	19	20	21	22	23	24	25	26	27	28	29	30	31	1	2	3	4	5	6	7
February	1	2	3	4	5	6	7	8	9	10	11	12	13	14	15	16	17	18	19	20	21	22	23	24	25	26	27	28			
Nov. / Dec.	8	9	10	11	12	13	14	15	16	17	18	19	20	21	22	23	24	25	26	27	28	29	30	1	2	3	4	5			
March	1	2	3	4	5	6	7	8	9	10	11	12	13	14	15	16	17	18	19	20	21	22	23	24	25	26	27	28	29	30	31
Dec. / Jan.	6	7	8	9	10	11	12	13	14	15	16	17	18	19	20	21	22	23	24	25	26	27	28	29	30	31	1	2	3	4	5
April	1	2	3	4	5	6	7	8	9	10	11	12	13	14	15	16	17	18	19	20	21	22	23	24	25	26	27	28	29	30	
Jan. / Feb.	6	7	8	9	10	11	12	13	14	15	16	17	18	19	20	21	22	23	24	25	26	27	28	29	30	31	1	2	3	4	
May	1	2	3	4	5	6	7	8	9	10	11	12	13	14	15	16	17	18	19	20	21	22	23	24	25	26	27	28	29	30	31
Feb. / March	5	6	7	8	9	10	11	12	13	14	15	16	17	18	19	20	21	22	23	24	25	26	27	28	1	2	3	4	5	6	7
June	1	2	3	4	5	6	7	8	9	10	11	12	13	14	15	16	17	18	19	20	21	22	23	24	25	26	27	28	29	30	
March / April	8	9	10	11	12	13	14	15	16	17	18	19	20	21	22	23	24	25	26	27	28	29	30	31	1	2	3	4	5	6	
July	1	2	3	4	5	6	7	8	9	10	11	12	13	14	15	16	17	18	19	20	21	22	23	24	25	26	27	28	29	30	31
April / May	7	8	9	10	11	12	13	14	15	16	17	18	19	20	21	22	23	24	25	26	27	28	29	30	1	2	3	4	5	6	7
August	1	2	3	4	5	6	7	8	9	10	11	12	13	14	15	16	17	18	19	20	21	22	23	24	25	26	27	28	29	30	31
May / June	8	9	10	11	12	13	14	15	16	17	18	19	20	21	22	23	24	25	26	27	28	29	30	31	1	2	3	4	5	6	7
September	1	2	3	4	5	6	7	8	9	10	11	12	13	14	15	16	17	18	19	20	21	22	23	24	25	26	27	28	29	30	
June / July	8	9	10	11	12	13	14	15	16	17	18	19	20	21	22	23	24	25	26	27	28	29	30	1	2	3	4	5	6	7	
October	1	2	3	4	5	6	7	8	9	10	11	12	13	14	15	16	17	18	19	20	21	22	23	24	25	26	27	28	29	30	31
July / Aug.	8	9	10	11	12	13	14	15	16	17	18	19	20	21	22	23	24	25	26	27	28	29	30	31	1	2	3	4	5	6	7
November	1	2	3	4	5	6	7	8	9	10	11	12	13	14	15	16	17	18	19	20	21	22	23	24	25	26	27	28	29	30	
Aug. / Sept.	8	9	10	11	12	13	14	15	16	17	18	19	20	21	22	23	24	25	26	27	28	29	30	31	1	2	3	4	5	6	
December	1	2	3	4	5	6	7	8	9	10	11	12	13	14	15	16	17	18	19	20	21	22	23	24	25	26	27	28	29	30	31
Sept. / Oct.	7	8	9	10	11	12	13	14	15	16	17	18	19	20	21	22	23	24	25	26	27	28	29	30	1	2	3	4	5	6	7

2003 →
2004 ←

28 - 2001
29 - 2002 4
30 - 2003 5
31 - 2004 6

When Are You Due?

Your estimated date of delivery is 266 days from the date of conception, or forty weeks from the start of your last menstrual period. To use this chart, track that first day of bleeding, then look underneath. That number will be your estimated due date. But remember, a healthy pregnancy can last anywhere from thirty-eight to forty-two weeks, with only about 5 percent of babies actually born on their due date.

Changes in the First Trimester

Here Come the Real Changes!

Hormones are now surging through your body, and the changes you are undergoing, even this early in your pregnancy, are monumental. Your heart is working harder, your blood volume is increasing, your breasts are growing and preparing for feeding the baby, your uterus is enlarging and moving, and your baby's neurological systems are forming. Let's have a look at some of the things you may be going through now.

Morning Sickness

It's almost impossible to describe morning sickness to someone who hasn't experienced it. But I'll try. Imagine the worst hangover of your life, complete with the urge to throw up and an overwhelming sense of fatigue thrown in for good measure. Now imagine feeling that way for three or four months. That's about how it feels to have a bad case of morning sickness. Except it's not just in the morning—it's all day long, with the nausea peaking often first thing in the morning and then later in the day, either in the evening or in the middle of the night. In addition to plain old nausea, I often felt as though someone had their hands around my neck and was squeezing just hard enough to make me want to be sick. Very unpleasant!

What makes pregnant women so nauseated? Part of it is hormones, part of it is the tremendous changes taking place in your body, part of it seems to be additional nutritional stress on your body, and a big factor is the additional bile collecting in your stomach. When your stomach is empty (as it is first thing in the morning), the feeling can be intensely awful.

Every woman's experience is different, and some women never even get morning sickness. There is no way to predict how bad your morning sickness will be, and a second or third pregnancy will often result in a completely different experience than your first.

However, morning sickness is not all bad. Studies prove that women who have had morning sickness go on to have mostly normal pregnancies and actually suffer fewer miscarriages than women who don't ever get it. So chin up! You may think you'll never get through the next few months, but somehow you will.

Tricks to Combat Morning Sickness

There are a number of tactics you can employ to combat morning sickness. Here are a few that have worked for me and women I know:

KEEP YOUR STOMACH FULL.
Many women find that avoiding an empty tummy is a good way to keep from feeling sick at any time of day—or night. This is where the old cracker myth comes in. It's believed that munching on crackers, particularly in the night or early-morning hours, will keep the nausea at bay. This is probably true, since crackers will soak up the bile and fill the stomach quickly. Personally, I can't stand crackers, and the thought of eating them when I was already feeling sick was completely unappealing. What worked much better for me was to keep an apple by my bedside, and every time I'd wake up in the night to pee I'd just take a bite out of that apple. Really sour ones like Granny Smiths seemed to be the most comforting. During the day, sucking on sour candy also seemed to do the trick. And of course that old standby ginger ale lived up to its stomach-settling reputation. Ginger tea can help, too.

USE PAPER PLATES.
True, this is wasteful. But in my first few months of pregnancy the thought of cooking food was so repulsive that I almost couldn't bear to be in my kitchen. And the sight of a dirty plate could make me retch. So a friend bought me a huge stack of paper plates, and this enabled me to eat in

my own house again. Pots and pans, of course, were another matter. Thank heavens for take-out food!

LIGHT SCENTED CANDLES, GET SOME AIR.
Your house (and of course, everywhere else you go, too) may suddenly smell terrible to you. Burn scented candles at home if this helps. Avoid stinky places. Open your windows wide and get lots of fresh air.

KEEP THE CAT BOX CLEAN.
I always keep the cat box in my house very clean. Yet, nothing smelled as awful to me during my pregnancy as the litter box. But because of Policedog Nose Syndrome I literally had to hold my breath while changing it, then rush out of the room afterward to gulp fresh air. Many times just looking at the box, even when it was clean, would make me gag. As we've already discussed, cat poop is not the healthiest thing for pregnant women to begin with (as I'm sure my body was trying to tell me), so be sure to wear rubber gloves every time you change the box.

TRY NOT TO TRIGGER YOUR GAG REFLEX.
Even putting my toothbrush in my mouth was too much for me some mornings, and I threw up a few times attempting to brush my teeth. But I didn't want to pass up brushing, because of the increased risk of gum disease for pregnant women. So a few times I just used mouthwash and brushed for about five seconds. By the same token, pass on the prenatal vitamins when you feel you absolutely can't swallow one. Better to keep your breakfast down than just have a vitamin in your tummy.

KEEP A FEW EMERGENCY PROVISIONS WITH YOU.
I felt like a freak carrying around ginger ale and Wild Berry Lifesavers everywhere I went for a few weeks, but it was a technique that worked for me. One possible cause of nausea is an overproduction of nasty thick saliva, and sucking on candy seems to thin it down. The ginger ale helped settle my stomach and made me burp up gas. Armed with both, I could face the world…barely! Through trial and error, you'll learn what works for you.

SNACK AT BEDTIME.

A snack at bedtime is almost always necessary to make sure the baby has nighttime nutrients. If you haven't eaten anything, the baby will just drain off your nutrients and make you feel sicker if you awaken. Keep snacks by your bed for middle-of-the-night noshing, and have high-protein foods like leftover cold chicken at the ready in the fridge.

TRUST YOUR INSTINCTS.

If something doesn't appeal foodwise, don't attempt to eat it. Listen to your body. Some people think morning sickness exists to keep women from eating things that are toxic or just no good for them in pregnancy. Whether you want to believe that or not, if your body says, "Come near me with that fish fillet and I'll upchuck," it may be best to eat the beef instead.

TRY ALTERNATIVE HEALING.

Herbs and homeopathy may be helpful for nausea. I had good luck with taking the homeopathic drug Ipecacuanha (9c, though some recommend 30c) when my morning sickness was at its worst. I also took Pulsatilla (200ck) when I became overwrought emotionally. However, before you take any herbs or drugs, talk to an herbalist or homeopath (or your midwife or doctor). Read the *Wise Woman Herbal for the Childbearing Year* by Susun Weed for more ideas on this topic. Acupressure wristbands which press the nai-kan points in the wrists, help some women.

DRINK ENOUGH FLUIDS.

Vomiting can obviously dehydrate you. Drinking as much clear fluid as you can—especially water—is good for your body and for your baby.

DON'T GET TOO TIRED.

Exhaustion makes morning sickness worse. Slow down! Accept help, and don't wear yourself out. Many pregnant women find they have to start taking more time off from their jobs—and their friends, lovers, and social engagements. Your body needs to rest and grow the baby. If you don't slow down on your own, you'll get sicker till you have to. Why let it get to that point?

IF SYMPTOMS PERSIST.

Most women find morning sickness slipping away anytime between the twelfth and eighteenth weeks. If you find that symptoms persist, it's important to see your doctor or midwife. You may be seriously dehydrated and, in a worst-case scenario, need to be treated in hospital with intravenous fluids. As a last-ditch effort to curb acute nausea, you may be prescribed medication.

The Need to Feed

Newly pregnant women seem to take one of two paths with regard to food. One is to develop a tremendous appetite. This is what happened to me: I just couldn't seem to get enough to eat. I would devour a huge meal and then be able to eat another just an hour later. It was quite astonishing! In part, this was because I found eating alleviated my all-day morning sickness. And I was just plain more hungry than I had ever been. Other gals, however, find the mere thought of food disgusting, so if they're vomiting up food and liquids, they may even lose weight during their early pregnancy. Obviously, this is not a healthy thing for your developing baby, so consult a doctor if you find you can't keep food down at all.

Food Cravings

Every pregnant woman seems to crave different things. The myth about pickles held some truth for me, as I found the sourness of a good dill pickle the perfect cure for nausea. What I loved even more while pregnant was anything orange-colored—fresh oranges, orange popsicles, apricots, apricot nectar, tomatoes, tomato soup, and cantaloupe, as well as more unhealthy orange things like peach ring candies and canned Chef Boyardee Spaghetti and Meatballs. I can only deduce that this craving was due in part to my body's need for folic acid, which many orange foods have in abundance.

My theory is, if there's no one doing the cooking for you, get sustenance where you can! As my pregnancy progressed, I started craving a wider variety of things, including salad, milk, and cold barbecue chicken. I continued to devour fruit, though, and have since learned that many women crave fruit while pregnant.

Policedog Nose

Most pregnant women develop a supersensitive sniffer. It's probably your body's way of detecting rotten or toxic foods, and you should always pay heed to Mother Nature's signals. Certain smells will probably make you want to heave after just one whiff. If these are smells of foods, don't eat those foods. If they're environmental, try to get rid of them or at least avoid them for a few months. For me it was Christmas trees, gasoline, raw fish, the cat's litter box, and anything cooking in my house. Luckily, the worst aspects of this will recede when your morning sickness does.

Atomic Titties

Forget PMS-type sore breasts. Soon you may experience the growth of what I term Atomic Titties. This means that not only will your breasts start growing, they will hurt like hell. I could barely stand the pain, and the thought of anyone else touching them, even gently, made me recoil in horror. This pain will subside somewhere in your second trimester, but your breasts will stay large. They are preparing for the work of breast-feeding later on and will soon stop aching. Whether they will ever go back to your previous smaller size is an altogether different question!

Fainting

You can avoid fainting by making sure your blood sugar level stays constant, getting up slowly, and not getting overtired. The one time I fainted was in my first trimester, when I forget to have an early-morning snack before heading out to have breakfast with my girlfriend. We were in the restaurant, waiting for our food, when I felt an overwhelming urge to put my head down on the table. Next thing I knew I was out cold! Besides scaring everyone in the restaurant and almost ending up in an ambulance (luckily I revived just in time to cancel the one they'd called for me), I learned a very valuable lesson in basic self-care while pregnant.

Sleeping

Some pregnancy books say that you'll only need eight hours of sleep a night. Don't believe them! Every woman I know needed to sleep an incredible amount in the first trimester. Why are you so tired? First, your body is producing a new human being from scratch, which is very hard work, as well as building the placenta that will nourish it for the next nine months. Second, you're coping with tons of hormones flooding your system, making you a prime candidate for the debilitating effects of nausea and emotional duress. A good analogy is to imagine that your body is doing a similar amount of work as it would if you were going mountain climbing—each and every day! You may need to sleep up to twelve hours a night, as well as taking naps during the day. And remember that this will not be uninterrupted sleep but is likely to be filled with trips to the bathroom and cramming down a snack or two. Only you can decide how much sleep you need, so don't let anyone tell you you're sleeping too much. Spending enough time alone just being calm and quiet is also really important, especially early in your pregnancy. As your pregnancy progresses, you may find that you need slightly fewer overall hours of sleep, but your days of sleeping through the night are likely over. A good preparation for the early days of parenting to come!

Peeing

Especially during your first and third trimesters, when the growing uterus presses on the bladder, you will feel a very strong and quite frequent need to pee. Don't hold it in, or you may get an infection. Keep your fluid intake up, even if you may be tempted to drink less water to slow the increasing number of bathroom trips you'll be needing to make. You'll have to pee anyway, so you may as well stay healthy.

What—Zits Again?

Just when you thought you were a real grown-up and finally rid of zits for good, you may find that you have them back again. Outbreaks can occur on the face, back, chest, even shoulders. Blame it on hormones, stay as clean as you can, and try to forget about it. Obviously, if you have a serious skin problem you should see a doctor, but taking any medications for acne during your pregnancy is probably not a good idea. My two-month-long bout of tiny pimples on my back and shoulders stoped as suddenly as it had begun, and I had wonderfully clear, soft skin for the remainder of my pregnancy.

Taking Care of Yourself in the First Trimester

Eating for Two

FOOD REQUIREMENTS.

One of the hardest tasks of a new pregnancy is learning how to eat properly. Some women are so busy throwing up that the thought of trying to eat better or new foods can be daunting. Indeed, sometimes just getting something down is the most you can accomplish. Yet, dietary improvement in the first few weeks is extremely important. Not only is your own body's need for certain nutrients accelerating, but this is also the time your fetus is developing its entire neurological system. Since lesbian pregnancies are necessarily planned, we have an edge over some straight women, who may continue bad habits for months before they really accept they're pregnant. Since we're living in two-week cycles, we can start preparing our bodies for pregnancy each time we begin trying to conceive. This means starting to take prenatal vitamins either while we're trying to get pregnant or immediately once pregnancy is confirmed. I'd recommend taking them while you're trying, but they can be constipating, so you may want to wait. Or you can take a prenatal equivalent with less iron to avoid constipation.

NUTRITIONAL FYI.

It can be daunting to look at the nutritional "requirements" that most books and doctors recommend. The amount of food you're expected to eat, can seem like more than you could ever consume. You may ask yourself how you could ever stuff down five portions of protein and five portions of grains a day. Well, the answer is that you won't always be able to, but it's good to see what is recommended and adapt that for your own body. It's best not to panic about meeting every requirement on the food charts you'll be presented with. Generally, if you eat a well-balanced diet, including lots of fruit and vegetables, then add on extra protein and dairy, you'll be okay. The best thing to do is listen to what your body tells you it needs—and what it wants you to stay away from. However, it's a good idea to review the following information so you can make informed choices.

THINGS YOU NEED TO EAT ENOUGH OF

- Folic Acid. Folic Acid is a very important vitamin for prenatal development. Most prenatal vitamins should have 0.8 mg (800 micrograms) or 200 percent of the recommended daily adult allowance. Folic acid is also found naturally in foods like cantaloupe, oranges, and dark-green veggies like kale. It helps prevent deformities like cleft palate and neural tube defects like spina bifida, in which the spinal cord grows outside the spinal column.
- Protein. For a pregnant woman, getting enough protein is probably more important than eating enough green veggies. This means about three servings a day of meat, fish, eggs, or cheese. It can also include tofu and other soy products. If you're a vegetarian, make sure you drink milk and eat yogurt, beans, seeds, and nuts. Talk to your health care provider if you're a vegan, as you may need special supplements. Eating enough protein builds your baby's tissues, and it will also cut down on your morning sickness.
- Calcium. Calcium builds the baby's teeth and bones, and you need about 1,200 milligrams a day. If you drink milk or eat other dairy foods, you should get enough. I craved cottage cheese, which made getting enough calcium easy for me. Calcium is also found in dark green leafy veggies, dried beans, and canned fishes like salmon and sardines.
- Carbohydrates. Forget all those special diets currently in vogue that disallow carbs. You need lots when you're pregnant, and the emphasis should be on whole grains like brown rice, nonprocessed breads, and beans and lentils.
- Vitamins and Iron. Eating a well-balanced diet with enough fruits and vegetables (especially dark green leafy ones), along with a good prenatal vitamin pill, will generally ensure you get enough vitamins. Many women don't get enough iron in their regular diet, but prenatals should help bridge that gap. If you're a vegan, you should make sure you get enough B12 from the supplement you're taking. Iron helps your blood carry oxygen to the baby. It's also been found that eating or drinking vitamin C–rich foods like orange juice will promote iron absorption.

FOODS TO AVOID.
Of course, it should go without saying that you won't be consuming any alcohol or drinking tons of caffeine while you're pregnant. The occasional cup o' joe probably won't do any harm, but decaf may be a better choice—or even better, switch to steamed milk in the morning. You'll be getting the calcium your body needs and still somehow feel you're getting your morning fix of frothy hot beverage.

Since alcohol crosses the placenta, most women know that not drinking is the only responsible choice during pregnancy. If you enjoy an occasional glass of wine or beer, especially as your due date nears, you probably won't be doing any harm to the baby. But if you want to make absolutely sure of that, you won't drink at all. Since heavy drinking during pregnancy often results in a debilitating condition for the child called fetal alcohol syndrome, call a counselor immediately if you suspect or know you may have an alcohol dependency problem.

Avoid anything you have the slightest aversion to. It's your body's way of protecting the fetus!

If you're a tea drinker, remember that black teas are caffeinated, so herbal teas are a better choice. If you must drink black teas, try not to leave the tea bag in longer than a minute. This will decrease the amount of caffeine that seeps into the tea. A word of caution, however: some herbal teas have abortificant properties and may cause spontaneous abortion in pregnant women. These include pennyroyal and blue cohosh. Check with an herbalist for more details.

There are also some foods to avoid that may contain parasites or pose a risk of otherwise poisoning the fetus. These include raw meat of any kind, raw fish (order vegetarian sushi instead), raw eggs in salad dressing, and soft cheeses. In your first trimester especially, avoid bitter foods like broccoli, brussel sprouts, and onions. Some doctors think also avoiding the skins of potatoes is a good idea, as they are thought to be slightly toxic.

EMPTY CALORIES.

There's never been a better time to purge yourself of a junk food habit. Most of the baby's important neurological development occurs in the first few weeks after conception. If you aren't providing good nutrients then, not only do you risk causing the baby damage, but he or she will drain off your resources in desperation to get them. This will cause you to feel even more sick than you might already, so do both of you a favor and eat well.

The Full Rubdown

Many women extol the virtues of massage while pregnant. However, you should receive massages now only from someone who is experienced in doing bodywork on pregnant women. This is because there are certain pressure points on the body that should not be worked while pregnant, as they can cause miscarriage. You should also tell anyone who does acupuncture or any other bodywork on you that you're pregnant. By the way, acupuncture can help some women with morning sickness or other symptoms of pregnancy.

Hot Tubs and Sauna

In other parts of the world, limited hot-tubbing and sauna use are relatively common among pregnant women. However, the common wisdom in Canada and the United States in that both are considered unwise. Your body temperatures may rise too high, which could bake the baby or cause you to pass out. One of the hardest things for me in getting pregnant was giving up my weekly visit to San Francisco's women's sauna. But at the gym after my regular prenatal swims I'd still dangle my feet in the hot tub...ahhhhh...

Exercise

Exercise may well be the furthest thing from your mind in your first trimester. You may find that even walking two blocks feels like a mile. But the more you can move your body, especially while getting some fresh air, the better. Yoga, swimming, and walking are all good activities, but women who are more athletically inclined or who have the energy for it can still partake in most of their prepregnancy activities.

Girlfriends...the Emotional and Legal Nitty-Gritty

I am the bio mom in our particular family. I was pregnant after the third try, but it took a long time to even believe I was pregnant. Because I didn't have any morning sickness nor many changes in my body other than exhaustion, it was hard for my partner to tell anything was different. Then when I felt the baby kick and she couldn't, she began to feel left out and to get tired of the mind consumption of the pregnancy. My point is, there is that short period when the nonpregnant partner will feel left out, but reality will soon sink in. For us, this happened at around three months when we went to buy the baby's crib.—Fiona

Pregnancy can make the partner of a lesbian become almost completely invisible. I had so many doctors and nurses assuming I was my girlfriend's mother—even though I'm only six years older than she is! It used to drive me crazy!—Rose

The stress that pregnancy can cause a relationship is tremendous. If you are in a newer relationship, be prepared for some major boat-rocking. If it's a decision you've made together as a couple, be aware of the stresses it can cause for even the best partnership. Most couples weather the storm of pregnancy very well, and many girlfriends become rapt with delight at the baby growing within you. They will attend every doctor appointment, carry your sonogram picture in their wallet, and be the person who cuts the cord at birth. Congratulations, you have the perfect second mommy or even dyke daddy by your side!

On the other hand, your girlfriend may not be an active participant in your pregnancy. This is a hard one. It can be extremely traumatic to feel pulled in two directions during your pregnancy. There you are, absolutely excited about and dedicated to the tiny being within. You want to talk about every little change you're going through, and you want to share your excitement and worries with the person you love best. If she's disinterested, it will be upsetting and isolating, and you will wonder how she can actually love you and not also love your growing baby. You may find yourself censoring your excitement so you don't alienate your partner with too much talk about the baby. This can feel necessary in order to keep some equilibrium in the relationship, but it can make you feel resentful and lonely.

At the same time, even the most dedicated girlfriend can feel a bit lost when you are so wrapped up in something she can't feel or see yet. The changes she may witness in you—throwing up, sleeping all the time, etc.—may be alarming to her. Where did her old girlfriend disappear to? Especially if the pregnancy is more your idea, or you don't live together, or the two of you won't be actively coparenting, she may wonder about her role in it all, or even if she'll have one. She may also fear losing you completely after the baby's born.

Because every situation is different, I can't really recommend any particular coping plan other than keeping communication between the two of you as open and honest as possible. Life is not static, and situations and people can and do change day by day. You may find that your partner becomes more interested in it all once the baby is born and she can develop her own relationship with the new little person in your lives. Or you may sadly find that the birth of your child is really the last step in a breakup that's been building for some time. Try to make sure that you have other emotional support throughout your pregnancy either way, so you're not caught short feeling alone during this tremendously exciting but demanding time in your life.

The Legal Nitty-Gritty

My "family" gave birth to our daughter Chloe last year. I am the biological mom, but my partner Anna and I are sharing coparenting (or is it triparenting?) with Chloe's biological father. We all live together in a house we bought. We are in the process of dealing with legal contracts to make sure that Anna is legally recognized as Chloe's parent in addition to me and her father.—Juliette

In the state where we live, there is no second-parent adoption available to lesbian moms. We've had to make sure that we created our own legal documents and agreed to stick to them, even in the event that one day we broke up.—Melissa

Legally, you will want to prepare for the birth of the baby early on in your pregnancy, especially if you are planning on coparenting with your partner. The National Center for Lesbian Rights (see Resources section) can provide sample forms to help you, such as coparenting agreements. As of this writing, there are eighteen states in the United States (as well as a few areas of Canada) that allow second-parent adoptions. If you live in one of these areas and plan to do a second-parent adoption, you should get the ball rolling right away so you can finalize it right after the birth of the child. Formalizing an adoption may require a home visit, several interviews, and an appearance in court, and it will cost about $2,000. Seeing a lawyer is the only way to proceed.

If you cannot or choose not to have your partner adopt your child, then you may want to consider using the NCLR coparenting forms to establish the boundaries of your relationship as co-moms. Of course, not everyone wishes to share their child fully with anyone else, even in the confines of a committed, monogamous relationship. If you are not planning on actively coparenting with your partner, you should at least designate a person (who may or may not be your partner) to raise your child if anything should happen to you. In some cases, a power of attorney may even carry more legal weight than a coparenting agreement under the law, so coparenting couples should consider this too. If you are a single mother, you should still designate a guardian. If a guardian is not designated in any of these cases, biological relatives will be more likely to be granted custody by the court system

> *Prior to inseminating, all women should see a lawyer to discuss issues about known versus unknown donors, second-partner adoptions, and advice with respect to their role and involvement as parents.*
> *—Kate Kendall, Director, National Center for Lesbian Rights*

should you die. The NCLR forms provide a good starting point in keeping your family safe under the law. You should certainly see a lawyer in your own home state or province to personalize them for your own particular situation.

Not to dampen your enthusiasm during pregnancy, but it's best to think ahead a bit to what could happen if your partnership ever broke up. The NCLR is seeing an increase in lawsuits, especially when the non-biological mother is denied any involvement with the child upon a breakup. It's not being fatalistic to prepare for this possibility before you get pregnant. For the sake of the children, it's best to have as much advance legal preparation as possible for this event, as unlikely as it may seem at the happy moment conception is confirmed.

You and Your Health Care Provider

Many women find that it is easy to be out to their health care provider, and they have been throughout their doctor-patient relationship. If you haven't been out to your doctor before your pregnancy was confirmed, he or she may assume you are straight. Do both of you the favor of honesty; it will most likely make your pregnancy easier. If you cannot be out to your doctor because of your job or where you live, or for any other reason, at least make sure you are comfortable with the level of care you receive.

It's imperative for the long-term respect of our families that we honor our agreements with each other. If we don't respect our families, the legal system certainly isn't going to.

—Kate Kendall

If you have a doctor who is blatantly homophobic or who makes you feel uncomfortable in any way at all, consider changing doctors early in your pregnancy so you can have continuity of care with the new provider. If you do not have a regular doctor, talk to friends or other mothers in your area to get a recommendation for a doctor. Don't let fear of homophobia keep you from seeing a health care practitioner during your pregnancy. Midwives tend to be easier to deal with than doctors, so if you will not see a doctor, perhaps a midwife is the right practitioner for you.

You may want to consider hiring a midwife regardless of what your doctor-client relationship is like. In many countries throughout the world, women routinely see midwives for care through their entire pregnancies. In North America, the relationship between midwives and doctors is still a bit shaky. But as midwives gain certification in many states and provinces, more women are realizing that having a midwife is a legitimate, woman-oriented approach to prenatal care and childbirth.

In fact, midwives were helping women birth their babies way before doctors institutionalized prenatal care and labor. Midwives focus on the health of mother and baby and don't believe in unnecessary medical intervention during pregnancy or birth. The word *midwife* itself means "with woman," which pretty much says it all. Usually women who are planning home births hire midwives, but even if you're planning a hospital birth, a midwife can be a powerful ally to have by your side.

My midwives, Deborah and Dana of Awakenings Birth Services in San Francisco, provided emotional and physical support and care throughout my entire pregnancy. They came to visit me in my home several times and spent countless hours chatting with me and my partner about the changes we were going through. Unlike the five-minute checkups I had at my HMO, the appointments with my midwives gave me a real sense of the baby growing within me and how to care for it—and myself. When I had a complete emotional meltdown at one point in my pregnancy, Deborah was there to hold my hand and tell me everything was going to be okay. During labor, both women made sure I was as comfortable and cared for as possible as the baby within me made its journey into the world. After the baby was born, they made daily, then weekly visits to see me and Frances to make sure we were getting along okay. It's a so much more holistic and loving way to birth a new baby—and a new mother—than a hospital birth could ever be.

There are midwives in every part of the country, but the standard of care and costs will be slightly different in each region. The services of midwives are generally not covered by any insurance company, but the $1,500–$2,000 typically charged by midwives is worth it. If you cannot afford this, ponder the services of a doula, a professionally trained woman who will support you during labor and often care for you afterward.

The best way to find a midwife is through word of mouth from other women. Unlike most medical doctors, midwives will spend time with you talking about their services before you hire them. This will ensure that together you make the best team possible for the eventual birth of your baby.

Medical Tests You Will Probably Have Now

Many doctors will give you an official pregnancy test, even though a home test has confirmed your pregnancy. This can be either a blood or a urine test. Other tests you will probably have on your first visit include both blood pressure and urinalysis (expect them every visit hereafter), a pap smear, a blood test to determine RH type and exposure to rubella, and most likely tests for STDs and HIV. You will be weighed and may be offered an early sonogram if you have previously miscarried.

If you see a doctor for any other reason during your first trimester, it is imperative that you mention to the doctor that you are pregnant, no matter what you are being treated for. Now is also the time to lay off any pain medications you routinely take, such as ibuprofen, which may be extremely harmful to the developing fetus. Talk to your doctor about how you can manage any chronic pain or illness you have in ways that will be safe for your baby.

Genetic Testing

WHAT IS GENETIC TESTING?
Genetic tests are given to the mother to determine if the developing baby is at risk for birth defects or genetic disease. These disorders can include Down's syndrome, muscular dystrophy, hemophilia, spina bifida, epilepsy, and cystic fibrosis. If you use a sperm bank, you may have already been tested for diseases like sickle-cell anemia or Tay-Sachs.

SHOULD YOU GET GENETIC TESTS?

Some women shy away from genetic testing on the basis that they're "going to have this baby no matter what." That's an honorable credo. However, it's my philosophy that the more information you have at hand, the better. When you have to work so hard at getting pregnant as lesbians do, isn't it better to know all that you can about your pregnancy and baby to be as prepared as you can be?

Of course, this is a highly personal decision, and nobody can make you take any tests in pregnancy that you don't want. Some doctors will insist on more testing if you're over thirty-five, the rather arbitrary age that separates what they consider "low risk" from "higher risk." Should you follow a typical prenatal examination routine of tests, however, these are some you may have done:

Chronic Villus Sampling—CVS

The test for CVS is generally optional; it is only given if the mother is older or has had a miscarriage or there is a known risk of genetic defects in the family. It is performed when the fetus is between ten and twelve weeks of age. CVS is, along with amnio, one of the more invasive genetic tests. Actual cells are taken from part of the placenta, either by a tube inserted through the vagina and guided by ultrasound or by a needle through the abdomen. There is a risk of miscarriage and a slight risk of limb or foot deformities of the embryo, since the cells collected are from that region of the baby. Results may be ready as soon as a week after test. You may also be able to find out the sex of the baby with CVS.

Sonogram, or Ultrasound

Ultrasounds have become rather routine in prenatal care, but it is still up to you to decide if you want the test. Ultrasounds are usually first given some time between the sixteenth and twentieth weeks, but if you have previously miscarried, you may have one earlier. In this test, high-pitched sonar sound waves are reflected off your organs, creating an image on a TV-like screen. What the technician looks for are the location of the placenta and basic information about the health of your growing baby—as well as how many babies are actually in there! Ultrasounds are also used to determine how far along you are in your pregnancy, but if you've conceived through insemination, you generally know to the day when this happened.

The usual procedure for an ultrasound is that you go into a special room, take up your shirt, lie on a table, and have your belly smeared with gooey gel. Then the technician presses down on your belly with a hand-held device called a transducer, and the image is transmitted to the screen. It's exciting to see the image of your baby for the first time, even if it does look like an alien! I suggest bringing your partner or a good friend with you to share this moment. It's one of the big ones! Usually you will get a Polaroid-type picture or two of the baby to bring home with you. One of Frances still hangs on the refrigerator. These special photos fade, but there is a way to ensure you have a lasting first snapshot of the baby. My photographer friends advise that you take your sono pix to a photo lab, have the lab take black-and-white photos of them, and develop them into real black-and-white prints.

Some people are down on ultrasounds because they feel they don't provide enough useful information and they may disturb the baby. While I certainly don't advise taking any unnecessary tests, it can be very reassuring not only to hear that everything is fine but actually to see a photo of your baby. Some women also find out the sex of their baby during their first ultrasound, but generally, if the test is done before twenty weeks, you will not be able to tell. I walked into my ultrasound excited to find out and never knew until the baby was born months later.

Keep in mind, too, that what a technician sees is open to interpretation—you may be told you're having the opposite of what's actually in there! In some countries, such as Canada, it's now uncommon for parents to be told the baby's sex, since too many people were told they were expecting one sex, ended up having the other, and were disappointed.

While there shouldn't be any pain when you get an ultrasound, I found drinking the amount of water they suggested beforehand very uncomfortable. I also felt intuitively that my baby did not like this sonar invasion, and I opted not to have another scan for the rest of my pregnancy.

If you have previously miscarried, your doctor may want to give you a series of early sonograms this time around. Midwives often recommend postponing any medical intervention for a few weeks and instead relying on blood tests to check in with the baby. Remember, you have the right to refuse any medical testing that makes you uncomfortable, for any reason.

Expanded Blood Test

An expanded blood test is offered to women in many states at about the same time as an amnio would be if it were required. The blood test is noninvasive and can present information on the likelihood of genetic diseases and other problems. If the test shows a cause for concern, your doctor will recommend an amnio for further testing. You cannot know the sex of your baby from this test.

Amniocentesis

Amniocentesis is another invasive test, often given to women who are over thirty-five, and/or women who get questionable results on their alpha-fetoprotein test, or who have a history of birth defects in their family or a history of miscarriage. It will generally be given between weeks 15 and 17. Before fourteen weeks of gestation, an amnio will come with a 2 percent risk of miscarriage, after that, the risk goes down to between 0.2 and 0.5 percent. It will be up to you to decide if having this test is worth a 2 percent risk of losing your baby, as the hospital will probably not stress this statistic.

For an amnio, a thin, hollow needle is inserted into the amniotic sac through the front of the abdominal wall, and a small amount of amniotic fluid is withdrawn and used for testing. Some women experience cramping when the needle goes in.

An amnio is not foolproof, but it is over 90 percent effective in detecting neural tube defects and even more accurate in detecting Down's syndrome and other chromosomal abnormalities. It will also detect the baby's sex. If you are under thirty-five, in good health, and have no family history of genetic problems, there is probably no reason for you to have an amnio. If your amnio shows cause for concern, you will probably see a counselor provided by the hospital who can talk with you about your options at this point.

7

You're Well into It Now!
Your Second Trimester

Welcome to your second trimester, which people are fond of calling "The Golden Trimester." Whether it's really golden or not I'll leave up to you, but the middle months do seem to provide enough of a break from the weirder moments of pregnancy to at least allow you to catch your breath.

By now, you're used to thinking of yourself as pregnant, you're not as scared of miscarriage, and you're likely to start showing. People have probably been telling you that you'll feel better now than you've ever felt in your life, but this may be just because after the difficulties of your first few months, you're likely to almost feel like yourself again.

While many of the discomforts of your first trimester do fade out about now, don't expect a sudden cessation of its worst symptoms. Probably a gradual lessening of morning sickness will occur during the fifteenth to seventeenth weeks, though some women keep waiting...and waiting...for this to happen. Women who say they woke up one day and suddenly felt great may be exaggerating a bit in hindsight. You'll certainly be feeling better, but guess what—there is a whole batch of new things to fret about! But don't worry; the second trimester is also the time to enjoy a renewed sense of energy and joy in your developing baby's progress. And the time to start deep-cleaning the house and getting

What's Happening in There?

Weeks 13–15 Your fetus has grown to a few inches long and looks like a tiny human being. It weighs only about three ounces, but it is already growing eyebrows and hair.

Weeks 17–19 Your baby is about five inches long, has well-developed fingernails, and weighs between four and seven ounces. You've put on enough weight that your belly is swelling out, and you will need maternity clothes to stay comfortable now. If you haven't already, you will soon feel the baby move.

Weeks 20–23 Believe it or not, your pregnancy is halfway over. You may be just starting to get used to this whole thing, but your baby is already six to eight inches long and may weigh up to a pound by week 23. The top of your uterus now reaches your belly button. Your baby's ultrasound photo reveals him or her to look like a small alien. Strangers may notice that you're pregnant now, so get used to the constant questions and comments that are just beginning to come your way. Your baby's genitals are distinct now.

Weeks 24–28 Congratulations! Your baby is now considered viable, which means it could be born and still have more than a 70 percent chance of surviving. It may weigh up to three pounds by week 28 and be over a foot long, and it is covered with vernix, a protective white, waxy substance. Your innie belly button may now turn into an outie. You will notice the little creature kicking more and more, perhaps especially after you eat or just when you lie down to go to bed at night. The baby can now hear your voice and your heartbeat. You continue to grow, continue needing to pee often, and may have trouble sleeping. For some women, though, this is a period of relative ease, a time when you may regain energy and have a renewed sex drive.

everything ready for the baby's arrival. Your due date will be here sooner than you think!

I found my second trimester to be a time for getting things done. Morning sickness was over, I wasn't so tired anymore, and I felt inspired to get everything in order for the baby's arrival. People frequently said things to me like "You've got lots of time," but I didn't listen, and I'm glad. The weeks will speed by and the last thing you want to deal with in your third trimester is running around all over the place looking for that perfect mobile. It's also more fun to start buying things and arranging everything now than to wait till the very end.

The Big Payoff

Before you read the litany of second-trimester concerns in the following pages, know that a great moment awaits you any day now: soon, you will feel a definite movement from within, and you will know that there really is a tiny baby in there! This first feeling of the baby's movements, called *quickening,* can happen anytime from around the fifteenth through the twenty-second week. You will probably feel a slight fluttering within, almost like a butterfly's wings would feel brushing across your cheek. At first, you might doubt that you really felt anything, or you might dismiss it as gas. But one day you will know without a doubt that what you felt was real. Congratulations! You have just experienced one of pregnancy's great milestones, and there's no turning back from here. Soon those flutters will be jabs and pokes at all hours of the day and night! The movements will still be too small for your partner or anyone else to feel, so it's private-party time for the next few weeks. But by the end of your second trimester the squirms and wiggles can be felt by others, so get ready for the barrage of requests to feel your tummy.

Physical Changes in the Second Trimester

> When I ask if I am fat, I really don't want to know. But when I ask if I am showing, remember, "thick" is the best word.—Tracy

YOUR BELLY BEGINS TO GROW.

The main physical change of your second trimester you will see is that your stomach will begin growing quite noticeably. If you packed on the pounds your first trimester, you may have already begun to grow a belly, but now is when your tummy truly begins to swell. This is when most women start needing maternity clothes and start showing. This is also the time when you may experience a very itchy belly. As your skin swells over your belly, hips, and back, you may feel incredibly itchy there. Scratching is not the best tactic to take, as you may damage delicate skin in the process.

If you have a partner, have her warm up some vitamin E cream in her hands and then slowly and sensually rub it all over your growing parts. After all, body worship is always okay!

Many pregnancy books warn against buying any special creams for the itching, especially ones that claim to prevent stretch marks. However, I found it a real treat to buy myself a special jar of vitamin E cream, which I rubbed regularly on my growing middle. It was much more creamy than plain old drugstore lotion, and buying some special stuff felt like a small but much-needed luxury. True, I was left with mammoth stretch marks anyway (which eventually faded a bit), but it helped my psyche, if not my skin, to use the cream. You could also try breaking open vitamin E capsules and rubbing that into your skin.

EVERYTHING ELSE IS GROWING, TOO.

Hair and nail growth is also affected by pregnancy. Your hair may turn thick and grow more quickly now, though it may not have the same luster after the baby's born. In fact, your hair may even fall out in clumps for the first few months postpartum! This is normal, since you will then be losing all the hair you didn't when you were pregnant. Your nails may need cutting more frequently while you're pregnant, since they're likely to grow faster too. As the ligaments in your middle stretch to accommodate the baby, you may experience pain in that region. Special support bands can alleviate the discomfort.

GAS AND BLOATING.
It's one of those scary true facts: pregnant women get bloated and frequently have gas. There's not much you can do about it other than, as the great kid's book *The Gas We Pass* states, "Fart Thee Well."

As they say, pregnancy is a full-body experience!

SLEEP.
The constant need to urinate that you experienced in the first trimester may pass by the middle of your second trimester—which is not to say that you won't still wake up a few times every night. What is more likely, though, is that because of your swelling belly, the main problem you have now will be finding a comfortable position in which to sleep. You will not be able to lie on your stomach any more! Many women find that it helps to place a pillow between their knees, or on their side or back for support, or to use one of those special full-body pillows to drape themselves over. A cushy down comforter wedged between your legs and under your stomach is also really comfortable. As you near the end of your second trimester, you may also want to begin sleeping more on your left side. This will alleviate pressure on your vena cava and aorta, which are two major blood vessels supplying blood to the baby. When you get into your third trimester, lying on your left side also can be a good way to prevent preterm labor.

Do whatever you have to in order to get a good night's sleep, whether it be sleeping on the couch or cocooning in a big down comforter. If it means sleeping alone much of the time, so be it.

LEG CRAMPS.
No one is sure exactly why pregnant women get leg cramps (some suspect metabolic imbalance such as calcium deficiency), but I can tell you one thing: They sure hurt!! They usually strike at night when you stretch

out in your sleep. Gently extend your leg out fully in front of you into a runner's stretch and and massage it, and it should pass, although a bad cramp can sometimes be felt well into the following day.

JUICY MAMA SYNDROME.
You may notice that you have as much vaginal secretion as you did in your prepregnancy days, or perhaps even more. This is normal, and you shouldn't douche or do anything other than stay as clean as you normally would. My midwife, in calling it the Juicy Mama Syndrome, assures us that it is normal and healthy. Of course, if you have any thick discharge or burning or itching, you should contact your doctor or midwife. You could have a condition such as a yeast or bladder infection, which can be treated even during pregnancy, so don't be uncomfortable. You should also empty your bladder as often as possible to prevent infection.

CONSTANT RUNNY NOSE.
I think I kept the tissue companies in business when I was pregnant, and you may also be wondering why suddenly you're such a giant snotball. Indeed, your nose may run a great deal when you're pregnant, and officially, this is called *rhinitis of pregnancy.* It is caused by the production of the same kind of hormones that are preparing the mucus lining of the vagina for the delivery of the baby, which gives you a nose on overload! You may go through a lot of tissues, but you may also find that you won't get so much as a common cold the whole nine months of your pregnancy, which was the case for me. If you see blood in the tissue after blowing your nose, generally this is nothing to worry about. Some women find that running a humidifier in their bedroom at night helps alleviate the sniffles.

HOT-BLOODED MAMA.
Because you have your very own space heater inside you now, you might find that even the most cold-blooded among you will no longer feel as vulnerable to lower temperatures and minor illnesses. This is partly due to the fact that amniotic fluid, in which your baby is parked, is a degree or two higher than your nonpregnancy temperature. Perhaps this is a way our bodies have of protecting our unborn children from disease. In my

usual nonpregnant existence, I was always the one who needed a sweater or an extra blanket at night, so I found this a great bonus of pregnancy. Do make sure you stay warm enough to ward off chills, however, and make sure to stay cool and well hydrated in hotter climates. You don't want to suffer the indignities of a cold on top of everything else you may be coping with, especially since you won't be allowed to take much beyond a Tylenol or two. If you do get sick, be sure to ask your doctor or midwife what kinds of medications they recommend.

LINEA NEGRA.
Many women, especially darker-skinned ones, will notice a dark line appearing around this time, spreading from the belly button to the pubis. This is called the *linea negra* and will usually disappear after you give birth, although mine never did. Why does it appear? Who knows—but you can chalk it up to hormones like everything else.

BLEEDING GUMS.
Many women experience some slight gum bleeding or irritation during pregnancy. It even has an official name—*pregnancy gingivitis*. I found it to be at its worst in the early months. Brushing regularly, especially before bedtime and after meals, should keep this under control, though you may need a softer toothbrush to do so comfortably. My dentist claims that she often won't see a regular patient for a year or two after she finds out she's pregnant, because usually she'll be too busy with the new baby to make it in. So make sure to at least go for a checkup and cleaning early on in your pregnancy!

VARICOSE VEINS.
About 40 percent of pregnant women get varicose veins, most often in the legs. They're caused by blood pooling in the veins as a result of increased blood volume, standing too much, hereditary factors, being overweight, or just plain bad luck. While you may not be able to prevent them, exercise when you can and try to keep your legs elevated while resting to minimize them. Some find that rubbing calendula cream onto their varicose veins reduces them. They disappear after pregnancy, but they may return with subsequent children.

MASK OF PREGNANCY.
Because of hormonal changes, your skin may be more sensitive during your pregnancy. Any exposure to the sun may result in patches of darkened pigment developing on your face, officially called *chloasma*. This struck me right across the band of my nose and made me quite self-conscious. Supposedly, it can come back after pregnancy, too, so lather on that sunblock. It may help to bathe in cooler water, avoid drying out your skin, and drink more water so you stay hydrated.

BRAXTON-HICKS CONTRACTIONS AND EARLY LABOR.
I'm including this passage on Braxton-Hicks in the second-trimester chapter even though most pregnancy books assume it is a third-trimester issue. My first Braxton-Hicks hit solidly in my twenty-first week, far ahead of any woman I talked to at the time. Better to know what's coming, I say! Think of Braxton-Hicks as your uterus's way of practicing for childbirth. They feel like a small series of lightning bolts or squeezing sensations in your uterus that can move on down to your cervix. They can range from hardly noticeable to slightly painful, and they can really scare you when you haven't previously experienced anything like them. Braxton-Hicks (named after the doctor who first formally documented them) are perfectly normal as long as they do not continue for more than a few minutes. If they get really painful or last longer, what some doctors and midwives recommend is to drink some water, lie on your left side, and relax. If they continue, you should call your doctor or midwife, as you could actually be experiencing early labor, which you would want to stop as soon as possible! Drinking eight glasses of water a day is a good preventative for pre-term labor.

SHORTNESS OF BREATH.
Because the baby is growing and pushing up against your lungs, you may experience shortness of breath, particularly when exerting yourself, even if you're just walking uphill. Press your shoulders back to open your chest up as widely as you can, and try to maintain good posture. Rest when you need to. It's irritating to feel like you can't breathe, but there's nothing much you can do about it. When your baby's born you'll be able to stride up hills at full clip again, I promise.

HEARTBURN.
As your uterus grows, it presses on the stomach, causing stomach acid to back up into your esophagus. This, combined with the already sluggish digestion of pregnant women, can cause heartburn, that burning sensation that spreads across your upper chest and even into your throat. You can take antacids for this discomfort, but most midwives won't recommend antacids since they can block the absorption of calcium. Fresh papaya or papaya enzymes are a safer remedy. Eating more frequent, smaller meals that don't overload your tummy will prevent heartburn, as this will stop your stomach from leaking acid fluid.

HORMONALLY SPEAKING.
While the horrible mood swings of the first trimester will taper off, your second trimester may continue to be emotionally volatile. The best ways of keeping yourself balanced are probably to ensure you eat well and get enough rest. Take alone time whenever you need it, cut back on your work and social schedules if you can, and all in all, just pamper yourself! It's amazing what taking a nice long bubble bath while reading a junky magazine can do to ease the spirits.

Shopping

The second trimester is the perfect time to shop for some things for baby. It is also when you will start needing maternity clothes.

Maternity Shopping for Dykes

Yes, by now, your normally baggy clothes are probably just a wee bit too tight for both you and your ever-growing belly. That means it's time to take the plunge into one of pregnancy's oldest and scariest traditions: shopping for maternity clothes. Some women refuse to buy maternity clothes and just wear really big sizes of their usual duds. But these will be way too big in the shoulders, sleeves, and hems. Maternity clothes let your belly breathe while keeping the rest of you in proportion, so it's worth investing in one or two true maternity outfits.

The mall nearest you may sport scary frilly and stretchy velour wear that you'd never consider in a million years. And why should you? There are much better options around if you just investigate a little. The old standby for many pregnant women has always been a good pair of overalls. This is especially the case for those dykes among us who may consider themselves a bit more on the butch side of the scale. But buy them big so they'll fit through your entire pregnancy. I am a small girl, and I bought what I thought were a laughably big pair, but by my eighth month even they were feeling a bit snug. Maternity jeans with a stretchy waist may also be an option.

Maternity clothes have come a long way, so there's no reason you can't be both comfortable and stylish, no matter what your fashion tastes are!

If you normally wear dresses, try some basic loose cotton frocks, or spring for a few maternity dresses, which you can wear with specially cut leggings. I found this very comfy. Smaller-framed women may also be able to wear many of their looser-cut prepregnancy dresses throughout most of their pregnancy, even though the belly may bulge out a bit. I say, let it show, girls!

Certainly, we each have our own sense of style, but keep in mind that loose-fitting, all-cotton clothes will keep you most comfortable during your pregnancy. Check higher-end shops like Japanese Weekend (who also have really comfy nursing bras) for more chi-chi outfits and discounters like Target for basic wear like leggings, T shirts, and pants. A good pair of Osh Kosh overalls may be your salvation, but don't totally write off your local maternity store—they may even have a few acceptable togs if you're willing to sift through the velour to find them. Check the Internet for maternity clothes if you feel too sluggish—or self-conscious—to shop in stores.

Taking Care of Other Business

Since you will probably be feeling pretty good during your second trimester, this is the time to take care of other preparations for the baby. Why wait till you're feeling tired and uncomfortable to fix up the nursery when you can do all that now and be ready? People teased me about buying diapers when I was only fifteen weeks pregnant, but I'm a girl who likes to be prepared. During pregnancy, that's a good motto to have! Go shopping now for some basic necessities like a few boxes of newborn diapers (don't buy too many, as the baby will quickly outgrow them) and other layette essentials. It's also a good time to sort through donations of clothing people have given you, clean out dresser drawers and closets, decide where you'll want to give birth and how, hire a midwife or doula if you haven't already, and think about what other items you'll be needing once the baby arrives. While you're at it, you may want to write up a will or power of attorney, ponder day-care options, think about coparenting and second-parent adoption options if you haven't already, and look forward to the accomplished feeling you'll get from taking care of these details now as your due date creeps ever closer.

Remember to wash all clothing and bedding items with a baby-safe detergent like Dreft before using them.

Baby's Layette

Don't go on too big of a spending spree until after your shower, and even then buy sparingly, as the gifts may continue to roll in. However, you will need a few essentials, and you want them to be ready for the baby's arrival. These include a few items of each of the following, depending on your budget:

- Three to four tiny undershirts or "onesies."
- Coveralls and sleepers.
- A few pairs of socks or booties.
- One or two sweaters or sweatshirts.
- Two to three hats.
- A coat or bunting bag for cooler weather.
- Receiving blankets.
- Bedding for the baby's crib or bassinet, if you're using one.
- Burping cloths.
- And, of course, diapers.

Whichever diaper variety you plan to use, make sure you have them in newborn size. As far as the big debate over whether to use cloth or disposable, consider your lifestyle and budget as well as saving the planet. If you're a stay-at-home mom, using a diaper service or cleaning your own diapers may be something you feel committed to. On the other hand, if you're like me and run your own small business and plan to take the baby along, do you really want your store smelling like dirty diapers all day? These are decisions only you can make, since you'll be the one changing those thousands of wet, stinky diapers. Don't feel that as a harried mom you also need to fit someone else's profile of political correctness. Do what you need to do to survive and keep the baby happy, too.

Some Safety Tips for Baby's Nursery

- Use a crib with slats no more than $2\frac{3}{8}$ inches apart and no corner posts. The crib mattress should fit snugly, and you should not use loose bedding or pillows.
- Keep the baby's crib away from the cords hanging from window curtains or blinds.
- Install a smoke alarm in the nursery.

Taking Care of Yourself in the Second Trimester

Your Piercings

Pregnancy is not the time to indulge in a new tattoo or piercing. In fact, it's better to remove many of your piercings now, especially your belly button piercing. Nipple rings may become uncomfortable as your breasts grow, and if you plan to breast-feed, it will certainly be easier without plugs of metal in the way. According to Ariel Gore, author of the very cool book *The Hip Mama Survival Guide*, it is also advisable to take out your labia or clit rings. Skin may stretch out and piercings shift, and you also may not be able to reach down there very well over your increasingly big belly to clean yourself properly. Since this area may also suffer some trauma in labor, you may want to avoid having the piercings get in the way or be uncomfortable for you while you heal. You can put a temporary filling of plastic fishing line or plastic rings down there while you're pregnant to keep the piercings open, but as Ariel writes, "I'd consider taking them out early and kissing those piercings good-bye...You can always get them redone after you've finished procreating—once you've experienced labor, the pain of repiercing will seem like amateur stuff."

Exercise from Here on Through Your Pregnancy

While many women find that their energy level remains high through their entire pregnancy, others are unable to do much of anything from the first trimester onward. Still others may feel fine one day and exhausted the next. Go with the flow of your body's rhythms without forcing yourself, and you'll feel better for it. On the other hand, trying to maintain at least a mild level of exercise is good for you and the baby, as this will increase your body's flexibility and introduce more oxygen to your bloodstream than you'll receive by simply lying about. While some days, simply walking three blocks can feel like a Herculean effort, you may be able to do a moderate workout on others. I slept most of my first trimester but went kayaking in my third...go figure! At least stretch at home on the days your energy is lowest—you'll stay relaxed and toned for the extra effort.

Stay as active as you can within reasonable limits. It's good for both you and the baby, and will keep you in good shape for labor!

As you move into your second trimester, the best choices for exercise are walking, swimming, prenatal low-impact aerobics, and yoga. Prenatal yoga is becoming an increasingly popular exercise option for pregnant gals, and classes are given both by private instructors and through medical establishments. Partner prenatal yoga is also an option you can explore if your honey wishes to participate.

Unless you're a pro athlete or have these activities approved by your doctor, the no-no's of prenatal exercise include running, scuba diving, horseback riding, skiing, tennis, and heavy weight-lifting. Contact-oriented sports, including karate, basketball, and football, are definitely forbidden. You should also stop doing anything that works your abdominal muscles.

Personally, I found swimming to be the best prenatal exercise. As your weight and bulk increases, moving around on land may become harder, but in the water, your whole body is supported. No matter how tired and crabby I felt before I slipped into the pool, after a half hour of gliding through the cool water, I left refreshed and relaxed. The baby generally slept the entire time, too, rocked by the motion of my body doing all those laps. It was a wonderful treat for both of us, and I wish I could have indulged more than the two times a week I was able to get to the pool.

Don't Slip Up Now

Arriving at your second trimester can mean that a lot of your worries about your pregnancy, including those of miscarriage, will be alleviated. When the AFP comes back normal, your morning sickness disappears, and you start sleeping a bit better, it can be tempting to discard some of the vigilance you were just getting used to living with.

But while it's important to relax and enjoy your pregnancy, it's also just as crucial that you not slip up now. Remember to eat well and get enough protein, vegetables, and fruits to keep your baby growing well and your own health optimal. Eating lots of fiber-rich grains and drinking lots of water will also help you avoid constipation and hemorrhoids. Keeping your caffeine and alcohol intake low (or better yet, nonexistent), taking your prenatal vitamins, resting enough, and abstaining from any recreational drugs is the best ongoing gift you can give your baby in utero.

Medical Tests You Can Expect Now

If you are having a low-risk pregnancy, you won't have many tests in your second trimester. You will probably have monthly visits with your doctor or midwife, where you will be weighed, your blood pressure will be checked, and your urine will be analyzed. If you're having a higher-risk pregnancy, you may have additional tests and monitoring, all dependent on where you are getting care.

AFP Blood Test

Perhaps the one test that can cause the most anxiety or relief in the second trimester for women who haven't had an amnio is the Alpha-feto-protein (AFP) test. This blood test, which usually has the best results when given between sixteen to eighteen weeks, measures the level of AFP in your blood. This protein, produced by the fetus, may appear in high amounts if there is a genetic defect such as spina bifida or anencephaly, a condition in which the brain does not close. A low-level reading can indicate Down's syndrome. The test is not foolproof, however. There are false positives, and the test does not find every genetic problem. Still, it's a good test to have since getting a good result can keep you from having more intrusive tests such as routine amniocentesis. If the results suggest a problem, another ultrasound or an amnio will probably be recommended. I'm not a big medical test taker, but I did have this one, and I was relieved when the results came back normal. Sometimes we all need a little reassurance.

Glucose Screen for Gestational Diabetes

Only about 3 percent of pregnant women are affected by gestational diabetes, but many more show increased levels of blood sugar. The worst thing about having this condition is that you may grow too big a baby for easy delivery—a whopper of ten pounds or more! A routine blood test is done by most doctors between weeks 24 and 28 so that if you do have gestational diabetes, it can be controlled. For the test, you'll have to drink a bottle of what tasted to me like flat orange soda. Not pleasant, but not the horrible concoction I'd been warned about. An hour later your blood will be drawn, and the results are usually known in a few days. Some hospitals will also take blood for anemia and STDs at the same time. You can help lower your blood sugar level by cutting down the amount of caffeinated drinks and junk food you consume and by eating smaller, more frequent meals.

Belly Check

To check the baby's growth, your belly will be measured externally from your pubic bone to the top of the uterus with a tape measure. The measurement in centimeters should correspond roughly to the number of weeks pregnant you are. This will be done at your monthly appointments, along with a check of the heartbeat.

Thinking About Birth

By your second trimester, you should have given a bit of thought to what kind of birth you'd like to have. Of course, one never knows what's going to happen in labor, but you should have a rough idea about where and how you'd like to deliver. Talk to your doctor, your partner, and other women your age who have recently delivered. Most important, listen to your heart. Only you can decide which experience will be right for you. All the ideas you have about what kind of birth you'd like to have should be written up into something called a "birth plan." Making your birth plan will help you formalize these thoughts and will provide a blueprint of your wishes for the hospital staff. Some considerations for your birth plan include whether you would like to have pain relief and what kinds you prefer, whether you would like to be able to move around during labor or be allowed to have a shower, whether you wish to have a routine episiotomy, and whether you would like to be allowed to eat or drink during labor. Your birth plan can also include a preference for who will be present, how long you'd like to wait to cut the cord, who will cut your cord (perhaps your lover or a good friend), what you would like done with your placenta, and information about lying in with your baby. You may also want to make it clear, if you plan to breast-feed, that you do not want the hospital staff giving the baby a bottle, as this can hamper early breast-feeding efforts. Your birth plan is best shared with your doctor or hospital staff before labor begins.

Different Places to Give Birth

HOME BIRTH.
My home birth was a wonderful experience, and it was totally manageable without pain medicine. It was very reassuring to be at home with the people I loved and trusted attending to me. The midwives were incredible in guiding me through the experience and gently welcoming my baby into the world. If you have no major complications during pregnancy, home is a natural place to give birth. You get to pace around your own home, have a shower or bath, eat what you want, and go for a walk if you're able. Even if you initially reject this idea, it's an option that you can reconsider as you get close to term. Many women who choose a hospital birth for their first child are more open to the idea for their subsequent deliveries, because they now know what to expect of labor.

HOSPITAL BIRTH.
Most women give birth in the hospital. This is due in part to societal pressure, since people generally assume it's safer to give birth there. It's true there is more medical equipment at the hospital, but that also means there is a greater risk of intervention there. Some women have great medical coverage and don't want to pay out of pocket for a home birth. If you do give birth in the hospital, make sure to outline beforehand what you do and do not want to happen to you during labor. Consider what is the most intervention you will accept, and what drugs you will want for pain, if any.

You may also be able to use the services of a midwife or a doula in the hospital, and I advise you consider this. A doula is a professional labor assistant who provides guidance and support before, during and just after childbirth. Doulas are trained to focus on the mother and help her with her experience. Often they can advocate on the mother's behalf and ward off any homophobic attitudes from hospital staff, as well as ensuring that you are respected as a couple and family throughout the birthing experience. Midwives also provide this service. When you are in labor it is very difficult to concentrate on anything other than getting through each contraction, especially if you want natural childbirth. Having a midwife or doula there to advocate for you in a hospital setting and help you deal with labor is very empowering.

To find a doula, contact DONA, Doulas of North America at (206) 324-5440 or www.dona.com.

BIRTHING CENTER.
Are you leaning toward a home birth? Would you like to be attended by midwives but still deliver in the hospital? Then a birthing center may be the right option for you. Some hospitals have separate wings with a less institutional setting, and some birthing centers are freestanding. Many have hot tubs, showers, and real beds. And if you're really lucky, your insurance may even pay for the experience.

The Birth Certificate

You should also be thinking about how you would like your child's birth certificate to be filled out. For your own protection, unless you are thinking about coparenting with the father of your child, it may be best to leave a known donor's name off the birth certificate. Having his name on the birth certificate adds legitimacy to his relationship to the child and will be used in court as proof of paternity if he ever sues for custody. In addition, in the United States, if the father's name is on the birth certificate, you risk getting stopped at the borders to Mexico and Canada if you plan to travel with your child. You would need a letter of permission from the father every time you cross a border. That could be a big problem if you lose track of each other and you need to leave the country.

If you are using an anonymous sperm donor, you will probably put "unknown" on the line where the father's name usually goes, or leave it blank. You will need to check with your local municipal government for the laws that apply to you.

Preparing a Sibling

How you tell your other children and how they react to the news of a sibling on the way depends on their age. Toddlers won't really understand much, even if you prime them with details long in advance. By the age of three, a child may understand there's a baby growing in Mommy's belly but probably won't get interested or jealous till the baby's born.

Older children will probably pick up on the changes in you and the rest of the household, so early honesty will be the best policy here. In some families, an older child may be included in family decisions about this or already know that Mom—or her partner—has been trying to get pregnant. Good communication will carry the day until the baby arrives, and age-appropriate books on new siblings or how babies are born may be helpful to read together. If children are going to be at the birth, they need to be prepared for what they are going to see and hear, and what the laboring woman may act like. It's advisable that there be a support person available just for the child or children present. Many hospitals have policies about children at births, so inquire before arriving. Many people think that witnessing a birth is not appropriate for preschool children, as it may be too upsetting for them. A couple books you might want to check out are *The New Baby at Your House* by Joanna Cole (William Morrow), and *Za-Za's Baby Brother* by Lucy Cousins (Candlewick Press).

What Your Partner May Be Going Through

It is during the middle trimester that your pregnancy becomes noticeable and therefore "real" to other people. If you have a lover who has been very much with you during this whole process, it may thrill her to see physical evidence that the baby is thriving. For a couple that has planned a family together, there may be no greater joy than to realize that your baby is growing and changing and will soon join you in the world. On the other hand, you just can't predict what the reaction of your lover will be during your pregnancy.

I have heard of women who entered the pregnancy very much as a team, and are still happily coparenting their children years later. Others had the same intention but drifted apart even before the baby's birth, leaving the biological partner solely responsible. Still other women don't plan on actively coparenting and somehow end up doing it. Some begin their journey to parenthood solo and are perfectly content to stay that way, while others may begin single and meet a new lover while carrying the baby or after its birth. For every woman reading this book, there will be a completely different story. That makes it hard to generalize about what pregnancy is going to mean for you and your relationship or potential relationships. However, I can almost guarantee that pregnancy will test and stress you as a couple, which, if you look on the bright side of things, will be good practice for parenthood!

As anyone who has been pregnant knows, the experience is so all-consuming that it may be hard to imagine that anyone else can really experience it with the same intensity you do. Yet for all your aches and pains, your joy and wonder at the new life growing within, it may be alienating for even the best-intentioned lover. They can't feel the stirrings of life within you, can't feel those hormonal shifts, can't understand your sudden psychotic need for chocolate. They only see you as you present yourself, looking normal but somehow strangely changed. These changes include physical ones, of course, but they also may include spells of hormonal hell and weeks when all you want to do is eat ice cream and watch bad television. Your partner may well wonder where the fun girl she knew prepregnancy has suddenly disappeared to...and wonder whether she'll ever reappear. Luckily, pregnancy lasts only nine months, and the joys of family life and parenthood last forever.

If Your Life Circumstances Change

> Unfortunately, the relationship with my girlfriend started to go downhill as soon as I got pregnant. I wanted someone to take care of me and while she was supportive of my desire to get pregnant, she was not there for me when I did. Being in such a relationship provided an emotional roller coaster for my entire nine months, with my partner threatening to leave almost monthly. She eventually did soon after my son was born. I'm not sure how I ever got through all that.—Frankie

There is no great time to lose a job, move cross-country, have a parent die, or break up with a girlfriend. But life has a way of throwing us challenges that we somehow usually manage to cope with. However, coping with big life changes during pregnancy is even harder, because you will already be dealing with emotional and physical stresses. Cures you can try for the everyday blues are exercising, keeping friends close by, finding a support group (these days you can even find online support groups), taking lots of baths, burning candles, writing in a journal, and learning as much as you can about the growing baby inside you. Of course, professional counseling may be the best way to deal with some of life's big heartaches, since the optimal state for your pregnancy is one of excitement, not stress, anxiety, or mourning.

Keep in mind from the start that very few of us have absolutely blissful pregnancies, since during those ten months (and the many months or years spent trying to conceive) you do not live in a bubble. Some pregnancies occur just as a loved one dies, and it will not ease the pain when well-wishers point out that your pregnancy is part of the great cycle of life and death. What will help is time, and taking care of yourself in the meantime to the best of your ability. Relationships sometimes fall apart from the strain of both trying to conceive and getting through the many trials of pregnancy. If this happens, know you're not alone, look for and create a different kind of support system for yourself, and know that things do seem to have a way of working themselves out in the end. Once your baby is born, your hormones will settle down, you'll be back in your (close to) old body, and you'll have a baby whom you love and who adores you. If things hurt now, life will start looking up again soon! And don't worry about your normal pregnancy mood swings negatively affecting your baby. I cried a lot during my pregnancy and, luckily for me, I probably have the world's happiest baby!

CHAPTER **8**

Sex and Self-Esteem During Pregnancy

If you've read other pregnancy books, you'll know that information on sex during pregnancy is scanty. Most books have a page or two of information and a few illustrations of positions for heterosexual intercourse. References to lesbian sex during pregnancy are basically nonexistent.

Desire

Mainstream pregnancy books report that while some women lose desire, others experience great sex—and even their first orgasms—during pregnancy. In some cases, this may be true. If you are one of those lucky women who feel more sexual during pregnancy or manage to maintain your normal sexual prowess, more power to you!

> *When the urge hit during pregnancy, I wanted it then and there. I even had the urge the day our son was born. But we were out in public at the swimming pool, so unfortunately, it didn't happen!—Justine*

> *During my first pregnancy, especially toward the end, my sexual desire really increased. It was really a great time. Both my part-*

ner and I were hoping it would be that way during the second pregnancy. Unfortunately, it wasn't. I guess it was just a different mixture of hormones that time!—Pauline

When I was about five months pregnant, an old male friend showed up and stayed for a few months until the baby was born. Sex for me was quite enjoyable with him, right up until the end!—Christine

However, from talking to many women during the course of the research for this book, it became clear to me that the experience for the vast majority of lesbians (and probably also straight women) is that sexual desire tends to dip.

Sex during pregnancy...what's that?!—Miriam

My sex drive disappeared entirely while I was pregnant. My first trimester was spent feeling nausea every night, so who'd want to jerk and jolt around! By the time the nausea finally left, it seems like my hormones were on a roller coaster and I was just too exhausted. In the latter part of my pregnancy, my doctor cautioned me against vigorous sexual activity. I had to laugh, given my nonexistent sex life!—Debbie

During the first trimester, most women experience some degree of fatigue and nausea. Morning sickness is not exactly the world's best aphrodisiac! Neither is the overwhelming sense that you must go to sleep, often during the early evening hours when previously you would have just been starting to consider sexual activity. Your breasts may ache, your skin may itch, and you may be broken out with acne. You may also be worrying about miscarriage and not wanting to threaten your tiny fetus with any rigorous activity down there.

My wife and I have always had a very active sex life. But what with me puking for the first four months and the bad smell coming from my cooch in my last few months, neither of us was really in the mood. Plus, I'd just had a miscarriage and didn't want to do anything that could even possibly hurt this one.—Julie

In the later months, your desire may ebb and flow as your morning sickness decreases, but you'll still be aware that somehow, there's more to you than there was before. Feeling your body changing or even the baby kicking inside you may make it hard to abandon yourself to the realm of uninhibited sexual pleasure. As you get bigger, you'll also feel more awkward in bed, and finding comfortable positions for sex may be more difficult. And to add to the confusion, while some partners may find your new body luscious, some lovers turn off completely just when you start to feel comfortable with your larger size.

Indeed, Anne Semans, coauthor of *The New Good Vibrations Guide to Sex* and mother to a young daughter, says the "biggest issue for all pregnant women is total loss of sexual desire." While she concedes that some women do find their sexual desire increasing during pregnancy, she says that in her capacity as sex advisor and writer she has yet to run across many women who have that experience. Says Semans, "In pregnancy, you're dealing with your own body's changes...it's hard to keep up your sexual self-esteem."

Sexual Self-Esteem

So what's a girl to do?

After spending so many years in the same body, it's disconcerting to watch it change so dramatically, so quickly. It doesn't matter how much you've longed for this pregnancy—it will still catch you by surprise in many ways. I needed a lot of reassurance from friends that I was still the same vibrant, attractive person they knew and loved, especially when hormones swept over me like some giant tsunami and turned me into a hysterical weeping creature. Your partner may love you lots, but she's going through her own changes with all this, so it's good to have support from outside the relationship to help keep you balanced. Make time to spend with friends, and encourage your partner to do the same.

Exercise, quiet time alone, and special activities with or without your partner will also boost your morale. Take baths, read poetry, go for a walk on the beach, buy yourself flowers—because you deserve it!

Your partner can help here, too. As you go through physical changes, your partner can let you know you are still attractive to her. Many pregnant women get shy about their bodies when they start morphing. Of course, some partners know there's nothing more sexy than a pregnant woman. Those breasts! Those hips! That curvaceous belly! That growing life within! Your girlfriend can help boost your self-esteem by lavishing you with praise.

Intimacy

My own sexual urges were greatest when I was about six months pregnant, but my partner wasn't always willing to oblige. At the end, she wouldn't have sex with me at all. I was frustrated and couldn't see what the big deal was. I think she was scared of hurting the baby.—Kristin

Most women still want intimacy, even if they can't handle full-blown sex. A general emphasis on *touching* instead of sexual gratification may help keep you close.

Well-known sex educator Susie Bright suggests that couples focus less on positions and advocates that pregnant women receive lots of "tenderness and passion" during their pregnancies, even if it means they're more passive about lovemaking.

Actually, I felt more amorous through most of my pregnancy than I did beforehand. I definitely felt more sensual and emotionally open to my partner.—Sharon

Your partner may be feeling like she's lost her best friend now that you're focused on your pregnancy. With all the attention lavished on you, she may wonder what her role in all this is. Even if she plans to be a full-fledged coparent, she may be feeling left out. The world will naturally see the biological parent as the "real" mother at this point. It may be hard for her to feel intimate when she's feeling alienated! Encourage her to share in the decisions about the pregnancy and go with you to medical appointments. If your partner is not planning to coparent the baby, she can still share intimately in your pregnancy. Talking about your feelings is a good way to find reassurance for both of you; often pregnant women, in their own excitement, don't realize how much emotional support their partners need, too. Do what you can to keep communication open and your relationship solid.

If your girlfriend is feeling sex-starved, the best thing she can do is cut you some slack—and masturbate. Semans suggests that girlfriends of moms-to-be "show the initiative without putting pressure on your partner." This could involve giving her a sensuous bath, or a massage, then leading her to the bedroom and showering her with attention. If she feels safe and loved, she's more likely to open up sexually, even if she's tired or not really in the mood.

Susie Bright writes eloquently about sex during pregnancy in the essay "Egg Sex" in her book *Susie Bright's Sexual Reality*. She claims no woman really loses all interest; we're just consumed by our emotional and bodily changes. Documenting her clit's growth during her pregnancy, Bright says that she couldn't masturbate the same way anymore, let alone make love in the same fashion.

"Your normal sexual patterns don't work the same way anymore," writes Bright. "Unless you and your lover make the transition to new ways of getting excited and reaching orgasm, you are going to be very depressed about sex and start avoiding it altogether."

Try Something New

Anne Semans suggests trying to think of sex in a different way during pregnancy. How to do this?

There's certainly plenty of room for experimentation, and now is a good time to drag out those books on sensual massage or tantra. Semans suggests that couples try reading erotic stories or watching porno together, if you're open to those activities, or maybe get into some "really hot mutual masturbation." Here are some ideas to try:

- Read sex guides like the *Kama Sutra* on different types of sexual and spiritual expression.
- Rent your favorite lesbian porn video.
- Give each other massages.
- Buy a new collection of erotic stories.
- Masturbate alone and together.
- Plan a romantic evening.

- Share a candle-lit bubble bath.
- Plan a surprise weekend getaway.

For the truly sexually adventurous, pregnancy and childbirth preparation present opportunities for expanding your sexual consciousness. Susie Bright even suggests thinking of birth as the ultimate sexual experience. While not a sexual activity per se, perineal massage is intimate physical contact you can share with your girlfriend.

Perineum massage, in which the pregnant woman is stroked in the tender area between the anus and vagina, is a wonderful way to prepare those tissues for stretching during childbirth. Massage will loosen the tight tissue there and help prevent tears during labor. Lie back on a couch or bed, spread your legs, and relax enough so that your partner can really work the area both outside and inside your vaginal opening. She should use warm olive or sweet almond oil, and move her hands slowly. It could be quite uncomfortable the first few times you try this, since being touched in this area may feel unfamiliar. Eventually you should be able to work up to a ten-minute massage every few days.

Orgasms

In comparison to having sex when I wasn't pregnant, I felt my orgasms were now more intense, but it took more work to get there.—Arlene

During pregnancy, you may notice a difference in your orgasms. Increased blood flow to all your sexual organs may mean that your orgasms are longer and more intense. Women who have previously been unable to climax may be able to do so now. Still others may find that sex is a bit uncomfortable now, as excitement builds quickly but orgasm stays just out of reach. Masturbation may be one way to relieve sexual tension, or you may find you want to shy off your own pleasure for a while and simply please your partner. Just make sure you keep talking about where you are, and try not to get too shy about your body and the changes it's going through. Easier said than done, I know!

Questions About Sex During Pregnancy

Here are some short answers to specific questions you may have about sexual activities during low-risk pregnancies. If you have a pregnancy that is in any way considered high risk, I would personally err on the side of caution and only engage in sexual activities that cannot cause any trauma to you or your baby.

IS PENETRATION OKAY?

Penetration with fingers is considered quite safe. Penetration with dildos is usually safe in low-risk pregnancies. As with all vaginal penetration during pregnancy, avoid vigorous, hard thrusting, and stop at the slightest bit of discomfort. Many women lay off penetration entirely toward the end of their pregnancy as the baby moves further down the pelvis.

IS IT OKAY IF MY LOVER LIES ON TOP OF ME?

This should not be a problem in early pregnancy. In later months it may be too uncomfortable for the pregnant woman to bear the weight of her partner.

As the pregnant woman grows, Semans urges couples to be more creative about trying different positions. The pregnant partner may be more comfortable on top, or you can try making love side by side.

Toward the end of my pregnancy, some positions got a bit awkward, but generally improvisation worked well. It helps enormously if you have a partner who is turned on by pregnant women. Mine was, and boy was I lucky!—Tammy

IS FISTING SAFE?

Fisting is the practice of inserting a whole hand inside a woman's vagina. Contrary to its name, the balled-up fist is not forced past the vaginal opening but is slowly and gently inserted. After the hand is inside, it is curled into a ball—hence the term *fisting*.

I would not recommend fisting during pregnancy. One doctor I asked about this said that the pressure on the greatly engorged blood vessels could be dangerous to the mother's health. If you are determined to be fisted during pregnancy, make sure you are with a partner whom you trust (and who knows your body!), go very slowly and carefully, avoid deep, hard thrusting, and stop at the slightest bit of discomfort.

WHAT ABOUT ANAL SEX?

Anal sex is also safe as long as you proceed carefully, avoid hard thrusting, and stop at the slightest bit of discomfort. Start small: a finger, a small butt plug, a slender dildo. Tristan Taormino, in her book *The Ultimate Guide to Anal Sex for Women,* writes, "It is safe to have anal sex if you are pregnant, although some women find that they cannot get in a comfortable position for anal stimulation." Taormino suggests that pregnant women be extra careful about preventing any bacteria from traveling from the anal area to the vagina. This includes being very fastidious about keeping sex toys clean. It may be prudent here to point out that the same holds true when you use the toilet, since any vaginal infections that may result are more complicated to treat while you are pregnant.

IS IT OKAY TO USE LUBE?

A water-based lube is fine for vaginal penetration. Remember: Never use oil-based lubricants in your vagina.

WHAT ABOUT BONDAGE, PIERCING, CUTTING, AND WHIPPING?

Even the most sexually adventurous women should curtail any practice that may be unsafe during pregnancy. If you cannot live without this type of sex play, always let your partners know you are pregnant, lay off the heavy stuff like whipping, and stop at the first sign of discomfort. Bondage is not a good idea, as it can constrict blood flow and cause cramping. Basically, you are playing at your own risk, and the risk of your unborn child. Be careful!

WHAT IF I GET AN INFECTION?

If you notice any burning sensations, discomfort, or smells during pregnancy, it is always best to get them checked out right away. Many symptoms may just be part of the discomforts of pregnancy, but if you have an infection, you will probably need treatment. *Of course, you should always make sure anyone treating you for this or any other medical problem is aware that you are pregnant.*

WHAT IF I GET AN STD WHILE I AM PREGNANT?

While STDs are never pleasant, acquiring one during pregnancy is even more awful, because most can do harm to the fetus. You may also not be able to treat the disease in the same manner while pregnant because of the toxic nature of the medications. It is therefore best to err on the side of caution while you are pregnant and engage in safer sex, particularly if you have a new partner. In the United States, you will be tested at least once or twice during your pregnancy for STDs, and it is a good idea to get these tests even where they are not required. Your doctor will discuss treatment options with you if you are found to have an STD.

WILL IT HURT THE BABY?

We didn't have much sex when my girlfriend was pregnant, mostly because of me! A twins pregnancy is considered high risk, and I was so worried that we might do something that would hurt the kids, despite our great OB/GYN's blessing to go right ahead!—Elise

Many pregnant women instinctively shy away from sexual activities that may harm the fetus. And, says Anne Semans, that's probably a good thing. "If you're worried about a particular sexual practice, don't do it," she says. "Now is the time to err on the side of safety. One good fuck isn't worth the price of a baby."

While it's true that the baby is protected within the uterus, there are a few sexual activities that you should definitely avoid. While cunnilingus is generally fine, blowing air into the vagina is a big no-no, as it can cause an air bubble in the bloodstream called an *air embolism*, which can be life-threatening to the mother. However, this is a rare condition and not one that will come about as a result of regular sex play.

Anything that can damage the cervix is off-limits, including rough sex of any kind, thrusting too-large dildos inside you, and aggressive fisting.

On the other hand, my midwife Deborah Simone, of Awakenings Birth Services, says that a good, hearty session of sex may be just what a pregnant gal needs once in a while. She recommends staying away from deep thrusting into the vagina but says that making love doggie-style with penetration of the pregnant partner from behind may have its beneficial aspects. "It's a great way to get your perineum massage," says Simone of this position.

> *Sexual desire accelerated for me during pregnancy, but because of a past miscarriage, my partner and I were very nervous about sex. We had lots of sex while I was pregnant, but it was much more gentle sex, with limited vaginal penetration. The pregnancy was so precious to us that we didn't want to do anything that might jeopardize it. We had no formal advice on this and certainly wouldn't have felt comfortable discussing this with our doctor.—Sharyn*

If you have concerns or questions regarding sex during pregnancy, it will probably be up to you to initiate a conversation with your health care provider. Very few physicians will be knowledgeable about the specifics of lesbian sex during pregnancy. For instance, if a doctor says "no sex," does that mean no penetration? No oral sex? No orgasm? Be prepared to ask explicit questions.

> *During the first trimester of my first pregnancy, I started spotting after an orgasm. I was put on oral progesterone and was told not to have sex. I didn't know if this meant only no penetration like in heterosexual sex, and I wasn't comfortable enough to ask specific questions of my doctor. So I ended up not having much of a sex life during my pregnancy.—Diane*

Instead of giving up on sex, empower yourself with some sex-positive information and support. Try your local women's health clinic, and if you don't find the answers there, check out the sexuality resources in the back of this book. While the organizations in the resource section may not have specific info on sex during pregnancy, they can offer suggestions on talking to your doctor about sex.

CAN SEX INDUCE LABOR?

> *Orgasm always seemed to bring on contractions for me, and on the advice of my doctor, I had to lie with my feet up against a wall until they subsided.—Lee*

You may feel some contractions after sex, especially toward the very end of your pregnancy. This may make you anxious that labor could be triggered by lovemaking. While it's true that some midwives tell their clients to have sex or at least stimulate the nipples to bring on labor, this can really only happen if it's time for labor to begin anyway. However, if you are having a high-risk pregnancy, you may want to abstain from most sexual activity during the last few weeks.

CHAPTER 9

Into the Home Stretch: The Last Trimester

Congratulations on making it this far into your pregnancy! The good news is that for the first time, the end is probably in sight, and the months behind you will be starting to blur. Was it really you who was puking into the toilet each morning and craving apricot nectar every afternoon? How pathetic it may all seem now!

I remember my last trimester as a time when everyone kept telling me how excited I must be, and all I wanted to do was to punch them out. Sure I was excited, but I was sick of pregnancy, I could barely move, and I couldn't even see my swollen feet, let alone my vaginal area. It's natural to become crabby toward the end of your pregnancy, especially if the weather's hot. In fact, you'll know labor is close when you have the strange urge to kill everyone around you. No joke! The week I went into labor I even called my midwife to ask if this feeling was normal. She assured me that it was, and that labor was near.

But what really sets your third trimester, defined as weeks 29 to 40, apart from the early months is that now your baby really starts to grow big. If you thought you were getting large in your early months, you'll be amazed at how much bigger you'll get now. How does skin stretch so much anyway?

Particularly in your last few weeks, your baby will be gaining about eight ounces a week, which you may experience as gaining about a pound a week. You may feel like there is simply no more room left inside you, and you'll have the symptoms to prove it!

What's Happening in There

Weeks 29–32 Your baby already has all the hair it will be born with. He or she is now about a foot long and can see enough to know whether it is light or dark.

Weeks 33–35 The baby is inhaling amniotic fluid to practice breathing, and you probably notice when he or she gets the hiccups. Your baby is gaining a lot of weight now and may be settling into a head-down position.

Weeks 36–40 Now you're finally in the home stretch! The baby is continuing to grow, and by the end of week 37 it is considered full term. Your belly will feel huge, your skin will be stretched to the limit, and you may become really cranky. Finally, your baby is almost ready to be born!

The best thing to do in your third trimester is to relax. If you're still working now, take some time off. Load up the freezer with food. Go for walks to keep yourself limber, but have friends help you out with errands.

As your partner's pregnancy progresses, you as a coparent will feel more involved. You may even get some of her pregnancy symptoms, such as nausea and backache, like I did. And when she hits month eight of pregnancy, you will be the most important person in her life because without you, she won't be able to scratch her toes or pick up a sock.—Karin

My belly got really big, and my partner and I would lie in bed with our hands on my belly just feeling the baby in there and watching her move.—Sara

Common complaints during this time include the shortness of breath and heartburn discussed in the second-trimester chapter. You could also be suffering from hemorrhoids, those dilated, twisted blood vessels in and around your rectum. If you notice pain or itching when you poop, you may have them. The best remedy for, as well as the best way to prevent hemorrhoids, is to try to keep your stools soft. Eat enough fiber and drink lots of water!

You may also notice that your energy level will swing from high to low day to day. Many women also experience a rush of energy in the very last weeks, which helps them prepare for the baby's arrival. You may be overcome with the need to hang curtains or put the changing table together. This nesting urge may be nature's way of ensuring that you'll have everything in order before the big day comes. Just don't overdo it too close to your due date. You want to make sure you have plenty of energy for your labor!

Taking Care of Yourself in the Third Trimester

Childbirth Classes

We were one of two lesbian couples at our birthing class. Nonevent. The biggest thing I got from the classes was helping to understand the changes the body goes through in labor and the effects of different types of drugs you may be offered so you can make an informed choice.—Betty

If the idea of attending a traditional hospital class surrounded by straight strangers pushes your comfort limit, here is an idea that worked in our community: ask your caregiver if she is willing to approach her other lesbian clients about a lesbian childbirth series. Voila! Your own cozy class and an instant support system!—Phoebe

Taking some sort of childbirth classes is standard fare these days. There are many different types of classes taught today, the most popular of which is the Lamaze method, or some derivative of Lamaze. This method, which acknowledges that childbirth is painful, focuses on natural childbirth with an emphasis on breathing to control pain, relaxing as much as possible, and being as informed about the birthing process in advance as you can be. Usually you take childbirth classes a month or so before your due date, so that the information you learn will be fresh in your mind when you start labor. You can also take private classes from a midwife (which is what I did) if you prefer to learn about these things in a more intimate setting with your lover. Talk to your partner, talk to your doctor or midwife, and think about what may be the best approach for you.

The experience of taking birth classes as a lesbian or a lesbian couple among straight couples may initially seem intimidating. However, in most parts of North America today, most people won't bat an eye at two women attending birthing classes together, unless you yourself make a big issue out of it. Your classmates may know or assume you're gay, or they may just think you are single and have brought along the friend who's going to be your birth coach. Or they may not think about it too much at all. After all, everyone at these classes is there for the same reason; they will all be apprehensive, excited, and focused on their own experience, just as you are. Like many aspects of pregnancy or parenting in general, birth classes may help build bridges between lesbians and straight folks. These classes generally focus on things such as breathing techniques, different body positions and/or medications to manage pain, and possible complications that may arise in any birth.

> My partner and I are taking the classes once a week for six weeks, and we are the only lesbian couple. We also stand out in other ways because my partner uses a wheelchair and we are expecting twins! So we are unique, but the other couples are completely unfazed by us, although I'm sure we're the topic of conversation away from class! But the good thing about being in a class setting is that questions are asked that I wouldn't think of. Also, because I want everyone at the hospital to know just who we are beforehand, so there will be no surprises on delivery day.—Jennifer

Problems That Can Arise Toward the End of Pregnancy

There are no firm statistics, but it's thought that one in four pregnancies in the United States and Canada may be considered in some way high risk. And up to 10 percent of these births may result in a labor earlier than thirty-seven weeks.

What makes a pregnancy high risk? Any of the following conditions is considered to increase the risk of something going wrong: spotting or bleeding, DES exposure in a woman's mother, constant or sudden high blood pressure (often called preeclampsia or toxemia, characterized by protein in the urine, swelling of the face and hands and/or rapid weight gain), problems with the cervix or placenta (including placenta previa, where the placenta blocks the cervix, often requiring a Cesarean), or premature rupture of the amniotic water. Women expecting multiple births are often also considered high risk. You may be monitored very closely throughout your pregnancy if you have any of these conditions, and you may even be put on bed rest during the last few weeks. This can actually make many of the discomforts of late pregnancy worse, and you may need additional help and emotional support during this time. Stay in close contact with friends, let your lover spoil you, and think about contacting a national organization called Sidelines (P.O. Box 1808, Laguna Beach, CA 92652, or www.sidelines.org) which provides support and even a buddy system for moms on bed rest.

One of the most common problems that can arise in late pregnancy is the threat of early labor. While your baby won't be officially premature if it's born after thirty-six weeks, and not all preterm labor leads to immediate delivery, you want to keep the baby in your uterus as long as possible up to your due date. If you start having contractions that persist for an hour or more, notice the baby moving less, bleed from the vagina, or suspect your waters have broken, call your midwife or doctor immediately. In addition, you should also let your health care provider know right away if you start getting severe headaches, blurred vision, sudden swelling of hands or face, abdominal or chest pains, vomiting or diarrhea, or fevers over 100 degrees.

Will My Baby Be an Alien? And Other Normal Anxieties

In the few short weeks before the baby arrives on the scene, I can guarantee that you'll be focusing more and more on the birth and less and less on the long months behind you. It's perfectly normal at this time to really conceptualize the size of the baby inside you and wonder how it's ever going to get out.

> I remember seeing the movies of actual births in childbirth class and thinking very strongly, with my hand on my swollen stomach, "I'm not doing that. This thing's not coming out of me that way. They'll have to think of some other way." Yeah, right!—Chris

Of course, somehow they all seem to get out, one way or another. You've probably had enough prenatal testing and poking and prodding from your health care providers to know at least the approximate size of your fetus. You probably know the baby's position now and whether its head has dropped down and into position for birth. Therefore, you may have some idea if you're at risk for a C-section, or whether your plans to give birth naturally are realistic. It's a good idea to finalize your hospital birth plans now, or to get everything ready if you're planning a home birth.

You may also be feeling anxiety about whether the baby is really as healthy as you've been led to believe. For example, all through my last trimester I worried about whether my baby would be normal. When people said I looked small for eight months, I'd worry that the kid would be abnormally tiny. When they said I looked huge, I worried I was going to pop a ten-pounder. My partner teased me that the baby's hiccups were actually the croaks of a giant green frog that would leap out at any moment. Far-fetched? Of course. But just the kind of things a very pregnant woman will worry about.

> Don't worry that your baby will turn out like an alien if you have an unknown donor. Even when they were about to do my C-section, I said to the nurse, "I'm a little worried about what this child will look like," and she told me not to worry, that he would be beautiful. And sure enough, he is.—Lillian

This Woman Deserves a Party

Your Baby Shower

Most showers are given during the third trimester, and many occur in the last weeks of a pregnancy. It is traditional for a friend or relative of the pregnant woman to throw the shower, but I have heard of women giving a shower for themselves. Why not? Every pregnant woman deserves a party, and a shower is the perfect opportunity to gather together all the important people in your life and rejoice in the expected arrival of the new clan member. For dykes, quite frequently this means that if you have only one shower, family members and queer folk will be bumping shoulders. Some women will prefer to have a separate family-given shower to avoid clashing cultures, but if you are out to an accepting family, there's no reason not to have a party that's a true mixer. Showers can also be a time, especially for single mamas, to get a real sense of commitment from friends to care for you and the baby in the immediate weeks (and ideally, months) after the baby's birth. You may want to put it out there that the best gift you could receive is the knowledge that your friends won't all disappear after the baby comes home!

Some people think that only women should attend a shower, but feel free to invite whomever you want, without relying on old, outdated traditions. The same goes for what actually happens at your shower. There is a whole list of games and activities that happen at traditional showers, but I found most of them so ridiculous for my circle of hip urban dyke friends that I vetoed all of them. Instead, I used the time to mix with and enjoy the company of my friends, many of whom I hadn't seen much during my pregnancy. There was lots of food and good conversation, and the party had none of the stress that might accompany a more organized affair!

Typically, showers are a way, especially for first-time moms, to receive often expensive goodies for the baby from generous friends. But if you're in the loop of hand-me-downs like I was, there's little you'll really need by the time the shower rolls around. Instead, concentrate on the celebratory nature of the day and revel in being the center of attention one last time—next time there's a large gathering, the baby will steal the show!

Shower invitations should be sent out several weeks in advance; list the time and place, as well as the host's name and phone number. Encourage people to RSVP so the host will know how much food to buy and how many people will be descending on her home. Saturday or Sunday afternoons are good times for many people, unless you are extremely religious or have a lot of sports buffs in your crowd. If you are using a registry, also list that information on your invites. Although some people consider any specific requests rude, I think it is better to let folks know if there are items you really need—or don't. For example, because I had already received several boxes of infant and baby clothes by the time shower day came around, I indicated that people should not buy any clothes smaller than one-year size. I couldn't bear to think of my friends wasting their money on items I would never use.

While few people can resist buying one or two teeny-weenie outfits for you, there are other more practical items you can express interest in, and many are almost cost-free.

Noncommercial Items That Will Ring Mom's Bell

- Shopping and cooking dinner for Mom during the baby's first month home. This is particularly a perfect gift for the single mama!
- Cleaning Mom's bathroom for about two weeks after the baby's born. This is a time when you can't bend over, you're still bleeding all over everything, and dirt anywhere will be bothersome. Oh, how I wished someone had offered to do this for me, but I was too embarrassed to ask. Eventually I hired someone to come in a few times, mostly to give my bathroom a good scrub.
- Coming over to play with the baby while Mom takes a good long bath—or nap.
- A gift certificate for or offer of an at-home massage.
- An offer to take photos of Mom(s) and baby, complete with developing double sets of photos.

After the shower, send out thank-you notes almost immediately, so that the task isn't hanging over your head in the short weeks before labor. You never know when Junior might make an early arrival!

What is a receiving blanket, anyway?

I figure the term must come from the fact that you "receive" the baby wrapped up in one of these, but who knows what its exact origin is. In any case, receiving blankets are those tiny blankets of cotton or other soft, breathable material that you will use to wrap the baby in, especially when they are newborn or you go outside. Receiving blankets not only keep the baby warm and are easier to use than putting multiple layers of clothing on a tiny, squirming baby but also are portable and easily stored in different rooms of the house or the car for quick access. They are also wonderful for swaddling the baby in, a very comfortable thing for a newborn used to the tight quarters of mother's womb. You will need a few of them, so stock up. You can use them for blankets in the baby's crib later on.

Further Preparations

Other Stuff to Have Around Before the Birth

- Maximum-size sanitary pads for postbirth discharge (called lochia) and bleeding. You will need these unless you have a planned C-section.
- Breast pads in case you leak a lot.
- A few packs of diapers—but not all in newborn size, as the baby will outgrow these very quickly.
- Rubbing alcohol and Q-Tips to clean the baby's umbilical stump
- A and D ointment for diaper rash, or a health-food store equivalent like Baby Bee cream.
- Mild baby soap and baby lotion.
- Baby-sized nail clippers—the baby's nails will be long and sharp!
- Bottles and formula if you plan to bottle-feed.
- Frozen food and bottled juice and water for you.
- Book on newborn care (I can take you only so far!).

Packing It Up

Even if you are planning a home birth, it's a good idea to pack a "hospital bag" containing both necessities and the items that might make your possible hospital stay more comfortable. My advice is to have this ready about a month early, so that you don't leave it to chance in the hectic flurry of activity that may accompany any sudden departure to the hospital. Don't forget to arrange for a pet-sitter.

What to Pack for Delivery:

FOR THE BIRTHING MOM
- Nightgown or comfortable, loose sleeping wear.
- Warm socks or polar fleece slippers to protect your feet against cold hospital floors.
- Bras (if you wear them) or nursing bras.
- Heavy-duty maxi pads for postdelivery bleeding.
- Hard candy to suck on during delivery.
- Eyeglasses, especially if you normally wear contacts.
- Lip balm.
- Your own shampoo and soap and soft towel.
- Trashy mags in case you need to stay a while.
- A clean outfit to wear home.
- Any insurance papers you may need.
- Any essential oils, like lavender, that you may wish to use.
- Candles and matches.

FOR THE OTHER MOM OR BIRTHING PARTNER
- Massage oil.
- Cassette or CD player if you want to play music (make sure batteries are working and music is loaded!).
- Camera or video with film already loaded.
- Coins for phone and phone numbers to call.
- Snacks, bottled water.
- A change of clothes.

- A swimsuit in case your partner wants you with her in the shower and you're not the type to get bare naked in front of a bunch of other folks.

FOR THE BABY
- A name...since most hospitals won't discharge you without filling one out on the birth certificate!
- A receiving blanket.
- Newborn-size diapers.
- An outfit to wear home, complete with a hat to keep the baby's head warm.
- A rear-facing infant car seat, as is the law in all fifty states.
- Your "baby book" if you want a handprint or footprint officially recorded at the hospital.

If You Are Planning a Home Birth

Very often your midwife will have you order a "birth kit" that is commercially prepared and available by mail order. These contain items for you like underpads, gauze, special homeopathic drugs like Arnica pills (200c) to heal post-birth bruising and soreness, and sitz bath, as well as items for the baby like a bulb syringe and newborn stocking caps. In addition, you will need to have towels and plastic tarps, sanitary napkins, and cleaning items like bleach.

It's also advisable to stock up on items like juice, ice, coffee, miso, and snacks that those attending the birth may want. Labor can sometimes take a few days, and three o'clock in the morning is not the time to realize that there's no food in the house. Have everything prepared according to the midwife's instructions and keep her phone number on your person wherever you go those last few weeks.

Make sure you have your phone list out by the telephone, that all your sheets and towels are clean (you'll go through a ton in the first few days), and that you know how to register your baby's birth in your particular city or town. You may need the midwife to sign papers or fill out a mock birth certificate at the time of the baby's arrival. Better to know exactly what you need to have before you schlep down to City Hall with the baby in tow.

The Circumcision Decision

Without the pressure to have a baby boy "look just like Dad," one would think that lesbians would have greater clarity on the circumcision issue than straight folks do. Yet while we abhor the practice of female circumcision in third-world countries, we remain largely ignorant of the practice we willingly perform on our own sons. I personally find this inexcusable. Circumcision is a largely unnecessary medical procedure that causes an infant great pain and has no place in the lives of our precious baby boys. Yet, large numbers of lesbians still have their sons circumcised, mostly because they are just following what they think is "normal" procedure. But if we are ever going to demand that society change its perceptions about what is normal or not, we should also look at the larger issues of child rearing and think how in turn we can change them.

Circumcision, which is performed on about 60 percent of American baby boys (but only about 20 percent of baby boys worldwide) is the surgical removal of the foreskin of a boy's penis. There used to be speculation that circumcision might prevent infections and penile cancer later in a boy's life, but the rates of these ailments are very low, and any boy can easily be taught how to care for himself and stay clean. Most childbirth educators and pregnancy book authors, as well as the American Academy of Pediatrics, do not recommend circumcision any more. Babies feel pain, and why any rational parent would subject a trusting young infant to this kind of trauma is beyond me. Please think carefully about this issue before deciding to simply follow in someone else's footsteps. And if you are Jewish and feel that circumcision is an important part of your cultural heritage, consider substituting some other ritual for the bris.

Last-Minute Legal Advice

If you haven't already followed up on some of the legal advice I've given you in this book, now is the time to do so. Although some legal agreements (like a second-parent adoption) cannot be completed until the baby is born, one thing you can do now is make sure you have a valid will. Many people never make a will; now that you are on the verge of parenthood, be a grown-up and get one done! Particularly since the law does not protect lesbians very well, a will can provide substantial proof of who and what is important in your life. It's always best to see a lawyer, but Nolo Press has published some good books on writing up your own will, with forms provided.

Before the baby arrives, have a will drawn up as well as any other necessary legal documents. I know that I had this huge fear of "What if something happens to me while I am giving birth?" I had already made my wishes clear to my mother and to anyone who would listen that if anything ever happened to me, the baby should be with my partner. But in a time of loss and crisis, I'm not sure what steps my Mom would take, even though she promised. I strongly recommend seeing a lawyer and making sure everything is taken care of, just in case.—Renee

Surviving Those Last Few Weeks

I think the purpose of the last month is to convince every cell of your being that you are ready for the next stage, even if it does mean labor and delivery of unknown type and duration, only to be followed by a little person for whom you have no idea how to care.—Jen

Ugh. My last few weeks were entirely uncomfortable. Most women who carry to full term or beyond find the last month a really difficult time. Not only does the baby go through a growth spurt in the last month, but it will also stay really active. Sleeping becomes very difficult, for not only can you not get comfortable, but you may wake up many times a night. I was up about four to five times a night to pee and was often extremely thirsty. I'd stagger to the bathroom, then slug down a few mouthfuls of water before going back to bed. Unfortunately, discomfort is something you have to endure if you carry to term.

My last month was miserable. I was huge, and the baby kept bouncing on a nerve at the bottom of my spine, which would cause me to yelp in pain at the oddest times. I peed constantly and lumbered everywhere. My mantra for the last trimester was

"I bend for no one." As for sleep...forget it! Didn't do it much for
the first six months afterward anyway—maybe that last month
was simply prep work for what was to come.—Sheila

This is also a tough time emotionally. You are so ready to meet your
baby, and so over being pregnant. And you may be on the edge emotionally. I was sick of answering questions about my very public pregnancy, and I thought some days that if I heard the questions "Do you
know if it's a boy or a girl?" and "Are you excited?" one more time I might
very well lose it.

Part of this was probably caused by lack of sleep, part by physical
discomfort, and part by real impatience to put these ten months of pregnancy behind me. My girlfriend and I were impatient for something—
anything—to happen.

Finding time to be alone may also become more important during
the last few days or weeks of your pregnancy. I had a sudden realization
that these were my last few days to ever really spend alone, and I cher-
ished the little bits of solitude I could carve out for myself. Whatever else
is going on, try to escape from people a bit if you can—go sit in the park,
or have a bath. There's nothing quite like lighting some candles, shutting
the bathroom door, and escaping into a bubble bath. What a great way
to chill out!

Things start getting very busy right at the end of a pregnancy. People
begin calling every day or so to see where you are, relatives may start
arriving to stay with you, and last-minute preparations are in full swing.
Yet, while you may want to stay busy and make the time go by, this may
be the time you most need peace and quiet. It's important to stay calm
and claim this time as your own, no matter how you want to spend it. If
you have a partner, try to enjoy this last bit of couple time by going out
for a special meal or treating each other to a massage. The more connected you both feel emotionally before going into labor, the better. If
you are sexually intimate these last few weeks, you may notice it's harder
to get into a comfortable position. You may also experience some contractions after orgasm, and your breasts may leak a bit. These are normal
occurrences, and they will not make you go into labor unless your baby
is ready to come. However, since nipple stimulation does release natural
oxytocin (which can be given as a chemical during labor to keep things

progressing), you may not want to do any extended breast play unless you're sure you're ready for the baby's arrival!

The Bitter End

Your pregnancy may have reached a point where you feel it is never going to end. You are at the bitter end now, but if you can just hang onto your sense of humor for a few more days, it will all be over soon!

The day before my baby was due I was feeling really cranky and ran into an acquaintance on the street. She told me the best ways to survive the last few days of a pregnancy were to drink lots of water, walk every day, and rent funny movies. I promptly went for a long walk through the park, then stopped by the video store and rented *GI Jane* and *Romy and Michelle's High School Reunion*. I rightly figured watching Demi Moore go through rigorous military training would make me realize that someone could indeed have it worse than I did at that moment. By the time I popped in the second film, I had lightened up, and I laughed all the way through it. That was definitely some of the best advice I'd received during my pregnancy!

As your due date nears, you'll wonder how you'll recognize the signs of impending labor, and what to do if all signs are go. Turn the page to the next chapter, and I'll fill you in!

10

Birth:
The Big Event

Is It Really Time?

The last few weeks have been hard, and by now you're really ready for this whole pregnancy thing to be over. But by the time you're feeling the most fed up, your body is starting to prepare for the inevitable, even if you're not aware of it.

One of the first signs that labor may soon begin is *lightning*, a fancy term for when the baby drops down deep and low in your pelvis. People may be able to look at you and be able to tell this has happened even if you don't feel it. Your vagina may feel bigger and softer, and you may also notice changes in your cervix as it softens and ripens for the baby's passage through. My partner checked me a few days before labor began to find that my cervix had moved down, was extremely soft, spongy, and flat, and she could insert a finger through it. It's normal to dilate a centimeter or two before real labor begins, and your doctor or midwife will be checking for this.

Another sign of impending labor is the beginning of persistent Braxton-Hicks contractions. You may feel these for months before your due date, but now you might notice them more and more frequently. Other signs include backache, weird cramps that make you feel like you're about to get your period, an upset stomach, or even vomiting.

When it comes right down to it, though, there are three surefire ways to tell if labor has really begun. These include passing the mucus plug, having your bag of waters break, and feeling the onslaught of real contractions. Unfortunately, not every woman experiences the first two, so you may be hot with contractions before you realize that things are really under way.

Passing the Mucus Plug

During my entire pregnancy, my girlfriend and I joked about the moment when the mucus plug would come hurtling out of me. Of course, this was a gross exaggeration of what we knew would happen, but we liked to kid around about it. The mucus plug itself is a gelatinous separator between the cervix and the uterus, and its appearance may mean labor is coming, because when the cervix starts to widen it will be forced out. However, some women pass this plug—also called *bloody show*—weeks before their labor starts, and others never see it, since it simply gets lost in the messiness of labor itself. Right when I was wondering whether my labor was starting, I went to the bathroom to pee and found that the toilet tissue was full of mucus that looked a lot like bloody spin. It was the indicator we'd been looking for, and seeing the plug was both a reassuring—and a terrifying—moment. Labor had begun!

The Waters Run Wide

Many women are anxious thinking about how and when their waters will break. Will it be at night, thereby soaking the bed? Or in the health-food store, in the crowded produce aisle? Or in the park, with small children gaping? There's certainly no way to know when and where, or even if indeed your waters will actually break. Women giving birth in the hospital may have their water broken to induce labor, while babies born at home are sometimes delivered right in their sacs.

What does it actually mean that your waters break? You already know that the baby has been kept safe in an amniotic sac for your entire pregnancy. When it's time for labor to begin, the sac breaks.

Despite the fact that we are trained by popular culture to view the breaking of the waters as a surefire, commonplace sign that the baby's a-coming, in reality, only a small percentage of women experience this in any kind of dramatic fashion. To be safe, place plastic sheets on your bed in case it happens at night, and if you're really paranoid, you could always wear a sanitary pad your last week or two. I decided to take my chances with fate, and as it turned out, the midwives broke my waters when I was already well into labor. Many women's waters do not break until contractions are under way, in which case you'll probably be at home or in the hospital anyway. It may come out in a sudden rush or trickle out, depending on whether or not the baby's head is blocking the flow of water. If your waters break early, don't panic, as amniotic fluid replaces itself every few hours. It is advisable, however, to check the color of the fluid itself. If it's got traces of brown or green in it, rather than appearing clear, it may have meconium (baby's first poop) in it, which could indicate a symptom of fetal distress. Be sure to let your doctor or midwife know immediately if your waters do break.

Most women go into labor in the evening hours, and most babies are born at night. Myth has it that this is because in prehistoric times, predators would see and therefore prey on newborn infants born in the day. If it was dark, the infants had a better chance of surviving till morning. Many people also believe more babies are born on the full moon.

The Contractions Begin

A typical labor may begin with contractions that come about every ten to twenty minutes apart, and last between thirty seconds to a minute. They will get longer and stronger and eventually come about every two to five minutes, until you hit transition. More on contractions and the different stages of labor in upcoming sections. Every woman has different kinds of contractions, and you'll know them when they start coming. Labor pain may feel as though your entire insides were shuddering, but the pain is actually centralized in your dilating cervix. It is assumed that contractions start far apart and that when they are close together the baby is about to come. I've heard of some women who do things like a bake a cake in between contractions. Ha! In my labor the contractions started pretty close together, and there was never much of a break in between. I could barely walk from the bedroom to the bathroom without having a contraction on the way there, and then another while I was on the toilet. Which, by the way, is a great place to spend some time during late labor, as it is almost a perfect birthing chair!

The Excitement of It All

It's best to make no promises to anyone about attending your labor. I told two of my best friends, one of whom is a photographer and was supposed to take pictures of my baby's birth, that I would call them as soon as I went into labor. Because I went into labor late at night, by the time morning came and I could have called them, I no longer felt it was the right decision. The midwives, my mother, my partner, and I had operated as a small, well-oiled team for hours already, and bringing anyone else into the equation felt wrong, especially in my tiny apartment. Labor is just too intense and surreal an experience to know how you're going to feel ahead of time. Of course, my friends were very disappointed. But it's your birth experience, so do what you need to do. It's the last time you'll get to make a purely selfish decision for a long, long time!

What's Labor Like?

I'm a single mom and had my best (male) friend as my coach. Wasn't it a hoot when he got to wear the "father" wristband! My labor was quick—just about four hours from start to finish. Hardly time to get settled in and get used to it. I kept my eyes closed during most of it so I could focus, but I'd look up and make sure my coach was there. I hadn't realized how much I'd need that comfort.—Stella

My labor room at the hospital looked out over a eucalyptus tree grove. I found myself swaying back and forth through my contractions, in time to the eucalyptus trees.—Paula

Because of the epidural, I gave birth on the hospital bed. My partner, Julie, held my left leg, and a nurse held my right leg, and as I pushed against both of them, our daughter, Ani, began to come into the world. With my first push there was a lot of excitement and activity, because Ani's head had crowned. She was all the way down the birth canal and just waiting for me to take her the rest of the way. Every time I pushed, you could see a little more of her head, and when I took a break, her head receded. They set up a full-length mirror so I could watch myself deliver, and it was the most amazing experience of my life, watching myself push and seeing her head come out more and more. We were chanting, "Come on baby, come on baby, we can do it, come on baby." And all of a sudden, literally, out popped her little head! Dark hair, round little face all scrunched up, the rest of her body still inside me. I heard Julie say, "She's here!" and no sooner had she said it than Ani turned her head toward Julie and opened her eyes to look right at her. It was unbelievable to realize that she recognized Julie's voice. We were both crying with awe and amazement!—Catherine

All the scariness melted away as soon as my midwife arrived and I felt like someone was there to support me. I found the contractions manageable and even though pushing the baby out hurt, it was an unbelievable feeling to finally welcome him into the world.—Mai

The pain didn't matter anymore, it was just everywhere and always. The last part of labor hurt me the most, because the crowning "ring of fire" is no exaggeration term! But some part of me was still coherent and listened when the midwife said, "Don't push anymore, breathe it out." I did breathe and after only a few more contractions suddenly I felt a big warm gush and then a squirmy wet thing was in my lap! I remember saying several times "I'm so glad it's over!" and crying before I realized the little squirmy thing was my baby.—Tamara

You may experience symptoms called *false labor*—or *practice labor*—anytime close to your due date. But practice labor's contractions will be sporadic and stop if you change positions. Believe me, when real labor begins, you will definitely know it!

For every woman, there's a whole different labor story. However, there are three stages of labor common to every woman, which occur before the baby is born and the placenta delivered. You may not really notice any differentiation while your labor is in progress, but in retrospect you probably will. If you have a hospital birth, you may be told you're in a certain "phase" of labor, but at home, the stages will all flow into one another. Here is a quick overview of each phase:

The Stages of Labor

First Stage

EARLY LABOR.
Many books advise to try to ignore early labor, but I found that impossible. How could I ignore throwing up while violent waves of nausea passed over me? Or a body that trembled with pain? Or the anxiety and excitement, beginning at 10:00 P.M. at night, when I realized my labor was actually starting? If this is your first baby, you probably won't be able to ignore early labor either. You can try to do the things people suggest for distraction, such as going to a movie, having a bath, or taking a walk. But my bet is that if you're like me and your contractions start with a bang, early labor cannot be ignored.

During early labor, many women think they have dilated farther than they have, and they go to the hospital only to be sent home till the next day. If you're having a home birth, you'll want to call your midwife now, but she may not want to come till you are further along. By the time my midwives came, I had already thrown up in the bathtub and paced the apartment for three hours, and I was approaching a hysterical state from not dealing effectively with the pain. As it turned out, I was already three centimeters dilated.

In early labor, which ususally lasts from six to twelve hours, the cervix is drawn up into the uterus and dilates (opens) and effaces (thins out). Of course, the first part of this can happen gradually over a period of days, but once you're about three centimeters dilated you'll know it's official. This is the time to eat something if you can, especially if you're having a hospital birth—you may not be allowed to later.

ACTIVE LABOR.
Active labor is when things really start to happen. This is when the cervix dilates from three to eight centimeters. You could be in active labor any-where from an hour (if you've had kids before) to eight hours (which is what a lot of the books say) to fourteen hours (which is about how long mine was), and there's no way to predict this in advance. The best thing you can do is pace yourself and settle in to this middle phase of labor. A hot shower may feel really good (my partner and I took one together that was about twenty minutes long!), and you may decide you're hungry. Although I did not want to eat during my labor, my midwife gave me gin-ger ale from a spoon to hydrate me and settle my stomach, and my part-ner fed me bits of fresh watermelon to nosh on.

During active labor, your contractions are coming two to five min-utes apart and lasting about a minute. They may have a peak in the mid-dle that is most painful. Mine were so bad that I had to hang onto my partner's neck, arms wrapped around her shoulders, head pressed against her chest. Just having someone's hands on me made the con-tractions bearable, and the almost constant back rubbing I received was a lifesaver.

The pain of contractions is not easily describable. It's not like break-ing your arm or stubbing your toe. It's not really like bad menstrual cramps, either. It's a lot more constant and intense, and it comes from a place deep inside you. The pain can easily overtake your entire being, making it hard to think clearly and be fully present. It can seem like this pain is all you have ever known and all you will ever know.

That being said, I can also honestly tell you that the pain of labor is a manageable pain. It is nothing to run away from. It is, as my midwife says, "pain with a purpose." Remembering to breathe as you've been taught in classes, or breathing along with your midwife or birth coach, will go far in helping you deal with your contractions. I found that walking around my kitchen was a good distraction; then I'd drape myself over the dining-room table and have a contraction there. I didn't stay in one position very long. You too should follow your body's leads and move as it wants to move.

Active labor, which usually lasts from three to six hours, may tire you out the most. It may feel like you can't do anything else but get through each contraction. You may start forgetting about the people around you and really begin focusing on your body. If you're in the hospital and considering pain relief, now would be the time to ask for it. Keep in mind, though, that once you have an epidural (a shot in the spinal column that numbs your entire lower body), natural childbirth goes out the window. If you do have an epidural, you may then need the drug pitocin to progress. Then you will be hooked up to a fetal monitor, you won't be able to move around at all, you will be flat on your back, and you will no longer be as active a participant in your own baby's birth. Some circumstances do call for medical intervention, of course—for example, if a woman's failure to progress in labor endangers the baby. But I would urge any of you who are considering a "routine" epidural to reconsider and put trust in yourself and your body. It's managed to grow this amazing life inside you for nine months, and it's probably also capable of giving birth to it just fine.

TRANSITION.

Okay, the transition time is when they say it really starts to hurt. Your cervix is dilating from eight centimeters to ten to let the baby's head fit into the birth canal. The baby feels very low and you feel like you want to push, but it isn't time to yet. I don't remember transition per se, but at a certain point when I thought, "I don't know if I can take this much longer," my midwives told me that I was already past transition, so I knew I could.

Many women get symptoms in transition like shaky legs, feelings of icy coldness or sweatiness, and irritability. And who could blame us? This may be when you yell at everyone around you, and lots of straight women curse their husbands for getting them pregnant. Of course, we can't blame anyone except ourselves for our condition, so we can't do that! Lots of gals decide then and there that they've had enough of all this and that they don't want a baby after all. I do have a distinct memory of squatting through a contraction, saying, "I've changed my mind. I don't want to do this anymore." Luckily, it was soon time to push!

Transition can last from a few minutes to an hour or more, depending in part on the position of the baby. Contractions during transition last about a minute, sometimes even coming less than a minute apart. It's very intense, but you'll soon be able to push, and the worst will be over!

Second Stage of Labor

PUSHING OUT YOUR BABY.

Finally, you can push! You're finally completely dilated to ten centimeters, and now is the time you'll finally be told that it's okay to push. After holding back in the earlier hours, it's a relief to many women to finally be able to do so. This stage of labor can last up to several hours for first-timers, but because you will be actively engaged in *doing* something besides dealing with pain, you will be excited and probably get a new surge of energy.

If your contractions are strong enough, you will feel the baby bearing down on your rectum. Like when you feel a big poop coming down, you will be unable to stop the overwhelming urge to get it out! Some women describe the opening of their body in this stage as a sexual feeling, but that wasn't my experience. For though it was intense, and extremely primal, it was painful. It was all about opening up as fully as possible to pass the baby out. I was sweating and had stripped naked. Wave after wave of pain would wash over me, and from the expression on my face, my lover could tell what was up and would ask, "Another one?" I was squatting through most of my contractions, exhaling deeply as I did so, and I found myself closing my eyes, bobbing my head from side to side, and moaning occasionally. Despite the screaming you hear about in birth horror stories, I found that tuning into a silent place deep inside me kept me focused, and I was afraid that losing it by getting hysterical would send me in the wrong direction. Many women grunt, groan, sigh, or moan during labor, and you should make whatever sounds come naturally to you. If you find yourself more prone to scream, try to take it down to a more guttural level, as this will be more helpful to you in giving birth.

Contractions come very close together now, often without a break in between. However, since you'll be working with the contractions now, they may not hurt as much. If your labor goes too slowly at this point, your doctor may want to speed things up with drugs like Pitocin. If you're at home, your midwives may give you herbs and pinch and rub your nipples. This pinching releases the natural hormone oxytocin, which encourages the uterus to contract.

The baby's heartbeat will be monitored very closely now to check for any sign of distress. This is because while it is difficult for the woman laboring, it is also stressful for the baby making his or journey out into the world. Particularly, all the pushing and bearing down you're doing can be hard on baby, and you may be given oxygen to supplement the baby's supply.

THE BIRTH.
You should now be in the place where you want to give birth, whether that's a birth pool, a bed, a hospital room, or your living room. For me, attempting to lie on the bed, a standard hospital pose, was an extremely painful thing. I much preferred squatting down through contractions while holding on to something—or someone! When I felt the baby really coming, I moved over to the foot of my bed. With one foot perched on the wooden baseboard and one foot on the floor, I spontaneously went into what's called a "crescent moon" position, leaning over into a kind of squatting arch. Nothing could have moved me from this position once I assumed it, and I found out afterward that this crescent moon shape is a position commonly and naturally assumed by women giving birth.

My partner supported my weight in front, the midwives were ready to catch the baby, and everything seemed to be happening quickly, loudly, and intensely. Then the baby crowned. When this happens, you will feel a burning sensation that some call "the ring of fire." I can see why. You feel absolutely stretched open, and it does hurt. At this point, many women in the hospital opt for a cut through the perineum, called an *episiotomy*, to enlarge the opening, but most midwives advise against it. After all, women have been birthing babies forever, and there *is* enough room for a baby to pass through, particularly if you have practiced perineal massage on this area or use hot compresses or oil during labor. Don't let any doctor tell you this is a "routine" thing that all women need!

By the time you feel the head crown, you've generally been through so much that you're ecstatic to feel it. That's because it finally means your baby is ready to be born! At this point, things happen very quickly. I remember midwife Deborah urging me, *"Push your baby out, Rachel!"* and then saying excitedly that she could see the head, and asking if I wanted to see it in a mirror. I said no, since I was seized with the incredible urge to just get that baby *out!* And I was holding my partner in a vice grip, begging her not to move, so she didn't get to see, either.

It was a spellbinding moment, riding this huge wave of contractions, feeling the baby coming. Then came the unbelievable, pure blind sensation of her hard little head moving out of me. She was just moving now on her own momentum into the world, and I could only ride it out. A second later, I felt her shoulders quickly push through, and as everyone was yelling "Here it comes!" the rest of her came tumbling out in a wet rush of goo. Then suddenly there was a baby lying face down next to me on the bed, struggling to breathe, making a tiny cry, and attached to my body by a long curly purple cord. My first, extremely eloquent, words upon seeing this wiggling, vernix-white-tinged but bloody little baby? "Oh my God, it's alive!" Brilliant, huh?!

Of course, your baby's birth will be completely different from mine. Maybe you're having a C-section, or perhaps you're delivering twins, or you've opted for some serious pain medication, or you have complications that require you to lie flat on your back, hooked up to lots of equipment. Whatever your experience, however, there will be that moment when you look at your baby for the first time and wonder at the miracle of birth. It sounds corny now, but it's true! You've managed to create this perfect tiny being, and you finally get to meet it. It's been a long time a-coming!

Third Stage of Labor

DELIVERING THE PLACENTA.
How anticlimactic! Yes, there is a third stage of labor. It is the passage of the placenta. By now the cord has already been cut, and you've counted

the baby's fingers and toes and watched as he or she was cleaned up, weighed, and given an Apgar test. This test measures the baby's color, heart rate, reflexes, muscle tone, and breathing rate a minute and then five minutes after birth. You've probably nursed the baby a bit, examined his or her hair color, and marveled at what a beautiful creature you've managed to create.

Probably the last thing you want to do at this point is push anymore. The doctor or midwife may press your abdomen to see if the placenta is ready, and this may hurt. You may be dealing with small contractions and bleeding. To quell the bleeding you may be given an oxytocin shot. But the placenta must come out, so after a few pushes, out pops this rather grisly-looking but miraculous organ that fed your baby. Because I was very sore and had a tear, birthing the placenta was unpleasant, but I was nonetheless fascinated by how this deep red and bloody "tree" had grown my newborn daughter.

The Incredible Placenta

All during your pregnancy, your blood passed across the tissues on the maternal side of the placenta to give nourishment to the baby, and the baby's waste products and blood passed back on the other side, to be processed by you. The placenta has also produced most of the hormones that ruled you the last nine months. And when it's time for the baby to be born, the placenta and uterus do a hormonal dance that, along with the baby's signals of readiness, triggers labor. Try not to be scared off by the "ick" factor and have a look at this incredible organ. The side of it that was pressed against your uterus is rough, and the side that was turned toward the baby is smooth and cushiony. It looks like a giant piece of liver.

Various cultures honor the placenta in different ways. Here in North America, most placentas get tossed in the hospital garbage, but you may wish to take yours home and bury it in some sort of ritual. Under a tree is a favorite place, I've heard. If I'd had a hospital birth, I probably would have left the placenta there, but my two midwives urged me to keep it. So I did, and it's still sitting in the back of my freezer, awaiting a proper burial. I'm sure I'll get around to it someday!

Dealing with Complications

Of course, not every birth goes so smoothly. Many women have complications of one kind or another somewhere along the way. This can include a failure to progress or even a need for induction, or problems involving the fetus, such as when the cord is wrapped around the baby's neck. However, most complications can be dealt with fairly smoothly by both midwives and hospital staff, so don't let the thought of what *could* happen stress you out beforehand. Each birth takes its own course, and you *will* be able to cope with whatever comes up along the way. Even if you have a posterior-facing baby and end up with the dreaded and painful "back labor," or have a breech baby and perhaps need a Cesarean, just remember that giving birth to your baby lasts only about a day, and after that you'll be able to enjoy the fruits of your labor for a lifetime.

> On the day we had our baby shower, five weeks before the baby was due, my partner said she didn't feel well. The next day we had a doctor's appointment, and once we got there our world went into a tailspin. They noticed a change in her blood pressure, and my partner's heart rate was accelerated. They put her on the fetal monitor and noticed that the baby's heart rate was dipping. Turns out the baby was breech, the amniotoc fluid had disappeared, and the baby had not grown for a month. That is when the doctor looked at me and told me we'd need an emergency Cesarean. They wheeled my partner into the emergency room and then cut away. I held her hand the entire time, while peeking over the screen to watch the operation. All of a sudden she starts crying that we don't have a girl's name picked out yet, but at the same moment the doctor pulls out the baby's legs and says "Don't worry about that, you have a boy!"—Erica

Partners Become Parents, Too

At the delivery you become a parent. One moment you're not and the next you are. The doctor will be finishing with your partner as you watch every move the baby makes while the nurses do their thing. You'll hover around the warming table and let the little hand wrap around your finger. It's an amazing transformation, just as profound for the person who didn't squeeze something that big out of a hole that small. How you got there is different, but once you're there it will matter very little to either of you. —Sonia

In a few weeks after labor, you will have lost most of the vividness of the inseminations and the pregnancy. But the parent feeling will be there, and you'll never lose it!—Randye

For the partner of the pregnant woman, the birth of the baby is also a moving, life-changing event. Although she probably won't be called "Daddy" in the birthing room, what she will experience throughout labor and birth will be very similar to what men in heterosexual relationships go through. She may not be able to feel the contractions, but she will probably be there to help the laboring woman get through them. I hung all over my partner during my labor, and her kind words, back rubbing, and general rock-solidness went far in keeping me focused, calm, and pain-free. This kind of support is wonderful to have in labor, and if you have a partner, it's nice if she can be the one to give it to you. Make sure she knows you appreciate her, because she's working hard trying to make you more comfortable!

Partners should focus on keeping the birthing woman comfortable in any way she requests or requires. Breathe with her, massage her, and be as upbeat and supportive as possible. Especially as she hits transition, stay calm and encouraging, don't freak out even if she starts to, and don't take anything she says or does now personally.

My midwife calls birth a transforming experience, and it certainly is for the partner, too. Any hesitations about sharing her life with a tiny baby usually disappear upon first glimpse of said child. Of course, getting through the birth may range from nerve-racking to a deeply spiritual experience for the nonpregnant partner. It all depends on where the birth happens, whether there are any complications, and how soon everyone can be together afterward as a family. Bonding will generally happen very soon for the nonbiological mama, especially since she isn't recovering from the rigors of labor. She may well take over the running of the household while you recover, and this can be a great relief to some exhausted birth mamas.

Now that you've become parents, how do you take care of your incredible little creature? There are lots of books about newborn care, and I recommend a few in the Resources section. You may feel stumped, but you probably know more than you think, as good sense and natural instinct go a long way in this parenting business. But turn the page for a few pointers, and then you'll be on your own very capable way!

CHAPTER **11**

Holy Cow, What Now?

The one thing on early mamahood I can say is, ask for other people's help and sleep when the baby sleeps. That's what the midwife told us, and boy was she right! Sleep when the baby sleeps.—Maria

Well, you've done it! Now you're well on your way to joining the proud ranks of lesbian mamas everywhere. Soon all this pregnancy and birth stuff will start fading from your memory, and you'll be wrapped up in the world of infants. Instead of obsessing with other women about ovulation kits and insemination timing, you'll be talking about how much your kid weighs and what kind of baby carrier you like best.

Keep in mind that your baby's first week in this world is a rather surreal time for both you and your baby, as well as your partner, if you have one. Your newborn is so tiny, he or she seems so fragile, and you wonder how in the world you'll ever learn to care for him or her. You're exhausted, and you're probably still sore and bleeding from the birth. You're still getting the hang of breast-feeding. Yet you feel full of love for your child and your partner. You've joined the ranks of families with children now, whether that makes you a family of two, three, or more. The miracle of birth is no small matter, and you'll be riding high on endorphins for about a week, so enjoy it before the hard work begins!

So saying, before I throw you out in the cold, I thought I'd better send you off with some new baby/mama advice. While there's way more to know than can be included in one chapter (see my list of recommend baby care books in the Resources section), here's some info that I could personally have benefited from having in Frances's early days.

What Is This Creature, Anyway?

As I said before, the very first words out of my mouth upon seeing my baby girl were "Oh my God, it's alive!" Another woman I know said, "Shit, it's a baby!" You may laugh now, but just you wait! Giving birth is strange enough, but seeing the creature you've nurtured inside of you for the last ten months is a revelation. And usually it's a revelation not of profound love (you're too exhausted—that'll come later) but of astonishment. What and who *is* this tiny thing, anyway?

Newborns are rather creaturelike, and they remain so until they're about five or six weeks old. They're squirmy and almost opaque in color, they can't control their limbs or eyes, and they seem unbearably fragile and otherworldly. They make pathetically tiny cries that sound like the cries of kittens, and you have no idea what the heck they want.

But all of a sudden, when the smoke's cleared and you're back on your feet, tromping around town with your little person in tow, you'll realize that your newborn is no more. Instead, you'll look down at your baby and realize that he feels a bit heavier and looks a bit longer. Good Goddess, are those rolls of *fat* on her little legs? And could it be that he's actually looking right into your eyes and *smiling*? And then you think about it a bit more, and you realize that you've become nonchalant and efficient at changing and burping your baby, and you've even gotten to be a pro at nursing. You know what all your baby's different cries mean, and you spend hours just gazing down at her sweet face, marveling at the hundreds of expressions she seems to make every minute.

Creature no more, your infant has become a sweet bundle of a baby, a real little person, and you've become a real mama. And now the fun starts.

But First...

Of course, before you get to that point, there are some questions you might have and some things you need to know. Here are a few of them.

Can I Love This Baby?

Of course, every woman's experience is different, but I'll bet if you did a candid poll of a hundred women, most would say they weren't passionately in love with their baby the minute it was born. For one thing, you're too tired! Giving birth might be the most physically and emotionally exhausting experience you'll ever go through, and all you really want to do at the end of it is rest. Think about it: for twelve or twenty-four or even thirty-six hours or longer you've thrown up, gone through contractions, been pacing your apartment or hospital room, haven't eaten, and eventually pushed your baby out. And at the end of it, just when you've finally gotten it out, and blood and who-knows-what-else is all over everything, there's this little creature squirming around and crying, and you're expected to be immediately bonded for evermore! I cried with joy when Frances was placed up on my belly, and a photo of us at that moment shows me looking both extremely emotional and extremely exhausted. But I can't say that I was absolutely in love. Bonding takes time, and true love needs at least a few weeks to deepen and grow. You're not a bad person if you don't feel like a mother right away. Soon you won't be able to imagine life without your child, and you'll love him or her madly. Allow yourself time to grow into the role of Mama, and soon you'll be wondering why you waited so long to become one. And by the time he or she is eight weeks old and grinning at you with sheer adoration, you'll probably be wondering when you can have your next one!

But What If It's a...?

No pregnancy book of all the ones I've scoured says anything about the disappointment of finding out, upon birth, that the gender of child you wanted ain't the one you got. And the only thing that even touches on it from a lesbian perspective is Jess Wells's extremely honest and tender essay "Born on Foreign Soil," from her collection, *Lesbians Raising Sons*.

Wells wanted a girl child so badly she paid to have the sperm "sex-selected" to better the odds of having one. When a nurse pointed out the baby's penis during her amniocentesis, Wells was devastated. She writes, "I had been planning on a girl. It was essential that I have a girl...I was profoundly disappointed. I wept. I sobbed to my friends."

Now sure, there may be some who read this section and say "Ungrateful wench! I want a baby so badly I wouldn't *care* what sex it was!" Well that's great, but some of us do have a strong preference for one sex or the other. Many, many lesbians would prefer to have a girl and just wonder what the hell they're going to do if they have a boy child. Others of us long for a boy and never in a million years expect to birth a baby girl.

I myself fell into the latter camp. I had always wanted a boy child, and I assumed that because of the mechanics of alternative insemination I would have one. During my entire pregnancy, all but two people looked at me and said, "You're having a boy." I also had bad morning sickness and pronounced hormonal mood swings, things I had heard were more likely to be caused by boys than by girls. Taking all this as confirmation of my hopes, I told everyone I was sure it was a boy, agonized in excruciating detail over the choice of a perfect boy's name, and plotted the perfect future my boy and I would have together.

Was I surprised when the midwife turned the baby over and we saw that what I had delivered was a baby girl? You betcha. As my eyes scanned down the baby's body, I quickly realized that this was the penis-free variety, and I wondered how this could have happened to me. Amid my partner's triumphant screams of "It's a *girl!*" my own heart dipped and dived in shock. How was this possible? Hadn't everyone said I was having a boy? Hadn't I wanted a boy more than anything in this world? *What was I going to do with a girl?!*

Well, there you have it. Hoping for one sex or another is a dangerous game, since you may well get the opposite. But take it from me...though you might be disappointed for a few weeks, and even have fleeting thoughts that you must be a bad person for feeling like this, soon enough this will pass. You'll feel blessed with the baby you got, so beautiful and happy and healthy! As my midwife says, you get the baby you're meant to have, and surely yours is the perfect baby for you.

So do I still want a boy child in my life? Yes, in some capacity, but I can't imagine life without my daughter now. I can honestly say that after living with her for only a month, I was hopelessly in love. It's been quite a while since I thought about the boy child that might have been. It's just me and baby Frances, and that's how it's meant to be.

As for Wells, in that same essay she remarks that a year after her amnio, she finds all her apprehensions about having a son "inconsequential." She writes, "My son is here. I am so in love with him and so bound to him that I would do anything to make his life joyous, healthy and safe."

And whether you hope to have a boy or a girl, no doubt you will feel the same way!

On Postpartum Depression

Your crashing hormones and the lack of sleep, coupled with real physical discomfort and the demands of a newborn, may trigger symptoms of postpartum depression. I'd say it's pretty common to have at least a touch of it. It hit me about a week after the baby's birth and lasted about five or six days. Lack of sleep was a major culprit in my feeling down, as was the bleeding and sore vagina. I couldn't believe no one had told me about the horrors of breast engorgement—or that I would feel so wiped out and sore that even walking to the bathroom would feel like a major insult to my poor body.

Women who have hospital births and are sent home without support tend to be most susceptible to the blues. If you've had a midwife attend your hospital birth or you birthed your baby at home, the midwife will most likely check in on you and the baby almost every day the first week. These visits, which become weekly and taper off at about six weeks postpartum, provide a wonderful form of support.

Hire a Doula

I like to describe the role of a doula as a professional equivalent to how women used to care for each other before the turn of the century. Mothers, aunts, and neighbor ladies all supported the mother in birth and then helped her afterward to keep the home running. Now we hire doulas to fill that role. It can be a real life-saver for a new Mom!—Arlene

If you haven't hired a midwife, consider hiring a doula to take care of both you and baby for the first week or two after your baby's birth. I have stressed this in previous chapters, too, and for good reason. Doulas are trained to care for new mothers and their babies. Besides cooking and cleaning for you, they can also answers questions about breast-feeding and make sure you're healing properly.

Of course, hiring someone to care for you costs money. Try to save an extra $200 or so for this postbirth care, and consider it an investment in yourself and your baby. If you can't afford it, organize friends to help you out, or at the very least stock up the freezer so you don't have to cook for yourself right now. If you feel that your sense of sanity is seriously threatened and you don't have much support, please call either a local organization in your town or a national one like the La Leche League.

Babies Bring Love—and Stress

There will be many times, especially when your infant is inconsolable, when you will feel like tearing your hair out. A lot of newborn babies cry often, and this can be very frustrating. Single mothers may especially grapple with feelings of being isolated and overwhelmed. When things get bad, the best thing you can do is pick up the phone to call a friend, preferably another mother. The other lifesaver is to simply change the scene. That is, put the baby in his front pack carrier and go for a walk, go have coffee, sit in the park, or head for a playground where other mothers will fawn over your newborn. Knowing when you're reaching your limit (and we *all* have one) and acting to circumvent feelings of anger at your newborn will help you both stay happy.

For Partners

If you're the partner of the birth mother, you're probably exhausted too, and both excited and scared about what this new being will mean in your life. Make sure you get your rest, and while you'll want to do lots for your partner, don't try to be a hero. If you can, line up friends and family or hire someone else to cook and clean, and simply be present for your sweetie and the baby. Instead of racing around doing the shopping, give your gal a foot rub, read her a story, or take care of the baby for a while so she can nap. You can always call up someone else and ask them to bring groceries by.

It's easy to get caught up in what chores need to be done, especially since a new baby seems to produce more laundry than an entire football team. Partners should also keep in mind that the birth Mom's crashing hormones may mean she'll be a bit nutty for a week or so as she adjusts to the demands of the infant and lack of sleep. Be as loving as you can, and know that Mom appreciates everything you do for her, even if she can't express it right now.

Your Body, the Birth Battleground

No one really tells you that getting a C-section is having major surgery. It's not like spraining your ankle. It was painful for weeks afterward. I'd rather go through a weeklong labor next time than have another Cesarean.—Lisa

I assumed I'd be back at work in a matter of days after the birth. Surprise! I would never have believed that I could bleed for weeks afterward. I had to learn that it takes time to heal.—Carlin

Some people may take offense at the analogy of your body as a battle-ground. But once you've had a child, you'll probably be able to relate. Whether you've had a Cesarean and are recovering from the stress of major surgery, or have had a vaginal birth, your body will never quite be the same. Your vagina is ripped and sore and the size of a football; there's blood everywhere, your tits are about to burst, your skin's flapping around on your tummy, you're severely sleep-deprived, and you're wondering if you'll ever be able to poop again. Sure, childbirth may be "natural," but there's not much that feels natural about bleeding for weeks on end.

When you are postpartum, there's nothing much to do about all this but relax and allow yourself to recover. Requiring you to stay in bed for two or three weeks may be nature's way of making sure you hang out with your baby. If all you had to do was pop it out and disappear, the human species could never have survived. There may be women, especially younger ones, who can have a baby and run a marathon the following week, but for the rest of us, healing takes time. The amount of time you need depends on your age, physical condition, and what kind of birth you had. The best thing I can tell you is to follow your doctor or midwife's orders, and don't try to push yourself. The last thing you want to do is hemorrhage or break open a tear (like I did) because you decide you must do laundry five days postpartum. Also, be very careful about how you shift around in bed. Just moving too quickly from one position to another can stress the delicate perineal tissue that can only heal if you stay still.

The right amount of time you need to recover from birth is as long as you need. Don't rush it or let anyone make you feel like you need to be superwoman. All you need to actually do is rest and be with your baby.

Keep in mind, too, that the swelling you'll have after a vaginal delivery will eventually go down. It may feel and look freakish down there for a week or so, but soon you will have your old body back—or close to it. Of course, there may well be a new skin flap or some scarring of sorts around your vaginal lips or perineum, especially if you have had a tear. This will be permanent, but it will likely recede or fade as you heal, so that it's basically unnoticeable. It's all just part of having a kid, along with possibly bigger hips and a squishier tummy. But do give your body a good five months or so to completely heal before you get depressed about what could be only temporary changes.

While You're Postpartum

Watch talk shows, have someone rent videos for you, read trashy magazines, eat healthy food, drink *lots* of water (this helps you heal and also to produce milk), take your vitamins, hire someone to clean your house (one of the best decisions I made!), and let yourself be treated like the queen you are. Try to take a shower every day, wash your hair, and change your clothes so you feel clean and fresh. Don't feel obliged to entertain visitors, don't worry if the dishes pile up, and don't fret about how in the world you'll ever raise this child. Just lie there and be with your baby. The rest will all fall into place soon enough.

The Milk Bar's Always Open

Breast-feeding has been an amazing experience for me. Sitting with my daughter, seeing little drops of milk at the corner of her mouth as she suckles, still gives me butterflies in my stomach. —Riley

Prior to my daughter's birth, I would never give myself quiet time to just sit, relax, and reflect. During our feeding sessions, there's little else to do but watch the beauty and perfection of my daughter. I enjoy this time together as much as she does!—Fatima

Breast-feeding is certainly the best choice you can make for both you and your baby. Best for you because it helps you bond with your baby, it helps your body heal faster, and it's cheap, always available, and a whole lot less fuss than formula.

The main reason to breast-feed, of course, is that it's best for your baby. Breast milk is the perfect first food. Your body instinctively knows just the right kind of milk to produce for your particular baby. It changes depending on your baby's age and even over the course of each feeding as rich hind milk comes in after the sweet first milk. Hind milk is richer in nutrients and also helps a baby poop.

Breast milk has natural antibodies that strengthen your baby's immune system, it helps prevent allergies in your child, and it may actually make your baby smarter than formula-fed babies. Breast-fed babies also get fewer ear infections.

Of course, there are women for whom breast-feeding may seem undesirable. Perhaps you find the thought of a baby latched to your breast too strange, or you may decide that bottle-feeding will make things more equal between you and your partner. Some women just don't seem to produce enough milk or simply find breast-feeding too painful. If you choose not to breast-feed, or you just can't do it, despite your best efforts, you're not a bad person. Formula will nourish your baby and promote his or her growth, just like breast milk does! But why not get your baby off to the best start you can and at least give breast-feeding a try?

Like many worthwhile things in life, breast-feeding takes patience and practice. It's a skill that both you and your baby have to learn together. Don't forget the La Leche League is there to help you, and they're only a phone call away. There are actually entire books written about breast-feeding, and I urge you to consult one of them for more complete information than can be included here (see the Resources section). However, what I can't emphasize enough is that the first step in breast-feeding is making sure that you and your baby are both correctly positioned. You should be sitting up comfortably in bed or in a chair with adequate back support, holding the baby close to your body in a position in which he or she is cradled in front of you. Then guide your baby's mouth toward your breast without moving forward yourself or slouching.

Some babies instinctually root around, heads bobbing, mouths wide open, as soon as they're put near warm flesh, like a cute baby bird waiting to be fed. Other babies have to learn how to breast-feed. To help such a baby, stroke her cheek to get her to turn toward you, then touch her chin or lip to get her to open up that little mouth. As soon as she does, jam the baby's head right onto your breast, making sure she has as much of your nipple and areola as possible in her mouth. If the baby just takes the nipple in her mouth, she won't get enough milk, and your nipple will soon be extremely sore. After a few days you'll know whether the baby's latched on properly or not by how she looks on the nipple (lips parted and smushed against your breast, nose pressed down almost flat) and by how the feeding feels. Burb baby after every feeding.

Most books will tell you that breast-feeding doesn't hurt. This is, unfortunately, not entirely true. The pain shouldn't be bad (this could indicate a problem such as thrush), but until your nipples toughen up, it will probably hurt when the baby latches on. When Frances latched onto my right nipple the first few weeks, I'd wince from the awful shooting pain running from the nipple up into my shoulder. Ouch! Luckily, that didn't last long. You could also experience cracking, blisters, and leaking, and you should consult your doctor or a lactation expert if you have any of these symptoms. My friend Jo said that when her son was born she would lie awake in the night nursing him, tears running down her face from the pain of it all. Unfortunately, this is a common occurrence, and at these moments you may think to yourself, "Oh, it wouldn't be that bad to bottle-feed." But if you can just stick it out, it will soon get better.

I admit to having given Frances a bottle of formula on two different occasions in the beginning. She was feeding every half hour then, and I thought if I had to put her to my poor raw, blistering nipple again I was going to scream in pain. A few days afterward, my nipples healed and hardened up, and that wasn't ever an issue again. After two or three weeks you'll swear you're getting the hang of it, and by the time baby is six weeks old, you'll wonder why you ever thought breast-feeding was hard. Why, you could swear it was the most natural thing in the world, and it feels good to boot!

The first few days of life, when your baby nurses she will only get small amounts of a premilk substance called *colostrum*. It's a thick, gel-like liquid rich in protein and infection-fighting properties. Colostrum also helps the baby pass its first meconium poop. Keep putting the baby to your breast, as this will help your real milk come in. This usually happens within the first five days of the baby's birth.

What no one told me was that with the arrival of your milk usually comes a horrible—albeit temporary—condition called *engorgement*. But I will tell you now as honestly as possible, without scaring you too much, that engorgement hurts. I didn't cry once during my whole labor, but I wept when my breasts got engorged. You will feel like two huge hard melons are sitting on your chest where your breasts used to be. This happens because not only are your breasts stuffed with milk but your body's sense of supply and demand is still out of whack. The only way to prevent losing your milk supply or getting an infection of the breast (called *mastitis*) is to get the milk out. To do this, many women use a pump they've rented or one that the hospital supplies. Having given birth at home and not being prepared for engorgement, I only knew something was wrong because the pain was awful and my breasts were too full for the baby to latch onto.

Instead of renting a pump, the midwife suggested that my lover suck at my breasts to drain them. It was definitely a bonding moment between my partner and myself to have her latched onto my poor swollen breasts, swallowing large mouthfuls of sweet, warm milk. If you and your partner are both willing to do this, it will be much easier than using a pump, not to mention cheaper and faster than renting one. Applying warm or cold compresses may also be recommended, though I personally found the cold much more of a relief. Keep a cold pack around just in case—or at least a pack of frozen peas!

As you can probably tell, there's a lot to learn about breast-feeding. But I can't emphasize enough that it's definitely all worth it. There's nothing like relaxing on a cozy couch, gazing down at the satisfied face of your baby suckling at your breast! It may be hard in the beginning, but if you can get through the first few weeks, soon you'll have your routine down, engorgement will be a distant memory, and your nipples will be all hardened up. It's a proud moment when you have gotten to this point and realize that you just might be able to do this for a good while more.

Breast-feeding may be "natural," but it is also a skill that both you and baby must learn. The early weeks can be hard, but it will get easier with time and effort!

A note about breast-feeding and fashion: It's possible to wear T-shirts and other everyday clothes to breast-feed. However, there are companies that manufacture clothes specially designed for easy breast-feeding. The clothes, mostly dresses and T-shirts, all have slits in them that you pull open and pop your nipple through. Especially if you're sick to death of maternity clothes like overalls, I highly recommend giving these clothes a try. Because nipples will often leak or spray when they get full, a good nursing bra is also a must. They support your heavier breasts and also absorb leakage. Bravado Designs sells black nursing bras—very comfy and stylish! You can contact Bravado at (800) 590-7802 or via their Web site at web.idirect.com/~bravado/.

The company I like best for nursing clothes is called Motherwear, which can be reached by phone at (800) 950-2500 or via their Web site at www.motherwear.com. Make sure to request their catalog—there's lots more in it than is displayed on their Web site.

For more breast-feeding advice, ask your midwife or doctor or call the La Leche League, an advocacy group that promotes breast-feeding. They can advise you over the phone at (800) LA-LECHE, or you can visit their Web site at www.laleche.org. They can help you find a volunteer in your neighborhood or town, which might be the best help available (and one I myself took advantage of) so don't be shy about contacting them...they exist to help support nursing moms!

If You Bottle-Feed

If you bottle-feed, make sure the formula you use has iron, don't heat the formula in a microwave (the liquid will heat unevenly and burn the baby's mouth), and don't leave the baby alone with a bottle propped up in his mouth, because he could choke! There's no reason bottle-feeding can't be as intimate a time as breast-feeding, providing you and the baby snuggle up and enjoy each other's company.

For the Partner

If you're the nonbiological partner in a couple raising a child together, the best thing you can do for your baby and partner is to encourage and respect breast-feeding. Help the nursing mom get comfortable, bring her a glass of water or juice, and help keep the mood mellow while the baby feeds. You may initially feel left out of the feeding process, but you can do your share by making sure you help your partner through the hard early weeks and find other ways of comforting the baby. Your partner will soon be able to express milk, allowing you to bottle-feed the baby, and in a few short months, you'll be able to feed the baby solid foods, participating more equally in the feeding process.

Will I Ever Sleep Again?

You won't sleep much for the first few weeks, anyway! The first week or two will be a time of difficult adjustment for the baby. Used to short cycles of activity and rest inside the womb, the baby will take time to get used to the outside world's schedule. Count on the baby sleeping in two- or three-hour segments at most in the early weeks, with several feedings throughout the night. It can wipe you out to not get enough deep sleep, but keep in mind that the worst of sleep deprivation will be over soon. If you have a partner, try to tag-team your sleep in the beginning so both moms get at least a few hours' worth. You'll soon learn to love afternoon naps. And remember to sleep when your baby sleeps. By the time Frances was six weeks old we were only waking for two to four brief night feedings and then getting up around 6:30 A.M. It felt absolutely luxurious!

What no one can really realize beforehand is how a six-pound baby can come home with you from the hospital and completely take over your life. You won't feel like you have time to do any-thing—even go to the bathroom—those first few weeks. It's over-whelming. Joyful, but overwhelming.—Timotha

On Attachment Parenting

Our son used to cry so much as a baby, we started bringing him into bed with us. He just seems to sleep better that way. And that means we sleep better, too!—Libby

Take a hint from native cultures who keep their babies with them all the time. We are mothers and it's our job to mother. Please don't think about having a child and then shoving it into a room by itself for the next eighteen years. Keep your babies close and they'll grow up, as mine has, to be happy, independent children with lots of self-esteem!—Alma

Get some sort of pouch to carry your baby with you on your body. They love it and you'll be more connected than if you just plop your baby in a stroller.—Anabelle

The idea of *attachment parenting* has been gaining popularity in recent years in North America. The funny thing is that what we have come to analyze and give a name to is actually how much of the rest of the world just naturally raises their children. Attachment parenting really just promotes the idea of spending lots of time together—or "attached." Generally, this includes breast-feeding, sleeping with your baby, carrying your child in a carrier or sling right on your body, and generally doing things a bit more low-tech than many parents do today. Most lesbians lean toward this style of parenting for their much-longed-for babies.

I found that attachment parenting was a natural fit for me. I loved carrying Frances in her sling, being with her almost every moment, and breast-feeding. But I did find that sleeping together all night was not possible for us after she was a few months old. When she was a newborn I loved sleeping with her. She slept draped over my body, often falling asleep at my breast and just staying there for hours afterward. Then when she was six weeks old, she got a bit heavy for that and began sleeping curled into the crook of my arm. By two months she slept by my side, a tiny person sharing my bed and my blankets, ready to greet me in the morning with a big, big smile. It certainly makes nighttime feeding easier and is a wonderful way to bond with the baby. And don't worry, unless you're on sleeping meds or have been engaging in drugs or alcohol (hopefully not, with a new baby to tend to!) you won't roll over on the baby!

However, by the time she was a few months old, Baby Frances was more aptly named Baby Windmill. Too much thrashing around during the night on her part meant Mama Rachel was getting even less sleep than she'd bargained for. It was a hard thing for me to do, but I cleared out all the stuff I'd stored in my family's heirloom cradle and finally put it to use. Now the baby usually goes to sleep in her own bed and joins me for a while during the night in mine. We both sleep better this way.

Especially as far as sleeping goes, do whatever you feel works best for you, and don't listen to all the naysayers who insist that sleeping with your infant will result in problems later. People have very strong opinions on cosleeping in the United States, so be prepared to hear a few no matter what you decide. Remember, you don't need permission from anyone to do what feels right for you and your baby. If your instinct tells you it's best for you to sleep—or not to sleep—with your baby, then that is the right decision for you.

The Beauty—and the Difficulty—of Becoming a Family

One of the sweetest times in my life was the period immediately after Noah was born. It was then that my partner and I realized that for better or for worse, we were now a family. All of the expense and work of trying to get pregnant and the whole diffi-cult pregnancy was now behind me. I had actually given birth to a baby! My endorphins buzzed, my hormones still flew high, and I was damn proud of the way I had labored and delivered my baby.—Judy

We broke up a month after Ryan's birth. It was just too hard on our relationship. Now I'm a single mom, and she sees him on Saturdays.—Val

Whatever kind of birth you end up having, try to enjoy the postdelivery period. Soon you'll be dealing with a parade of visitors, your body will be a wreck, and you won't sleep for weeks. You may also find that your relationship with your partner will now go through some tough times. The initial euphoria may give way to a time of tension as you work out your new roles as parents. Whether you're coparenting with your girlfriend or not, there will probably be a shakedown as you both figure things out. Remember that straight people have these same problems and that it takes time to grow a family. But being queer, we have the freedom to create new kinds of family situations, without the rigid boundaries straight married couples face.

If you're in a couple relationship, it's a particularly important time to keep the lines of communication open between partners. Don't stop talking about the changes you and the relationship are going through. While you might be the kind of lesbian who craves the white picket fence and an absolutely equal coparenting situation, others may want a less traditional arrangement. Perhaps the biological mom wants the majority of the control, with a part-time mama backup. Or it could be that Mom doesn't even know what she wants yet, and it may take some time for it all to work out. If you're a single mama it could be that your circle of friends or relatives will be your family. Whatever the case, expect a period of adjustment, and expect to be able to navigate it. Do keep in mind, however, that having a baby is a bit like throwing a bomb into the middle of your life. You can't just pick up and carry on as things were before. And unfortunately, some couples just don't survive the explosion. But you've come too far now for me to present you with any worst-case scenarios. So enjoy what you have today, and worry about the future tomorrow!

> *Only you— and your partner, if you have one—can decide what kind of family you want to create. Remember that a family can be created in all kinds of ways, and that families grow and change with time.*

Basic Baby Care

Fortunately, your little one won't care how much or how little you know; they only need to know that you're there for them. My first words to my daughter, after "I'm so glad you're here," were "Well, I guess we'll figure this out together." And we did.—Robin

You're almost ready to head out into the wonderful world of lesbian mothering. Soon, instead of reading pregnancy books, you'll be perusing baby and child-care books, but here's some sage advice to close. There are many volumes chock-full of information on how to take care of your baby, but in actual fact, the needs of your newborn are really quite simple: to be fed, changed, and loved, to sleep, and to be held as much as possible, preferably close to your body. You will have to learn your baby's cues and how to care for her, which can seem daunting in those first early weeks. But let me reassure you, much of being a good mama is instinctual, and the more you go with the flow, the easier things will be. Don't be afraid of your baby. If your baby is full term, he or she has already made it through nine months of life and is ready to be with you. The best thing I can tell you is to take in "expert" advice, mix it with what your heart and gut tell you, and most of all, *enjoy* being a mother.

Well, you've come a long way since the early chapters on mucus and pee sticks! Soon you'll be holding your newborn baby, a sweet, strong-willed, small package of amazing resilience, personality, and love. Sure, there will be tough moments, but nothing that you, a lesbian who so badly wanted a baby, can't handle. Your dream is coming true, so good luck—and remember to have fun. It's been wonderful to stand behind you during your journey to mamahood, and I'm proud to have been part of this process. I wish you all the joy and happiness in the world. After coming this far, you certainly deserve it!

12

Resources

BOOKS

NOTE: Check your local independent bookseller for these titles, or order from the author's bookstore, Bernal Books (415) 550-0293 or bernalbks@aol.com.

Lesbian-Specific Books

While there have been books other than the ones listed below written about the lesbian/gay parenting experience, these are the best of what's in print.

Challenging Conceptions: Planning a Family by Self-Insemination by Lisa Saffron, 1998. Available from the author: Lisa Saffron, Box 55, Greenleaf Bookshop, 82 Colston Ave, Bristol, England BS1 5BB. A British lesbian perspective on pregnancy.

Considering Parenthood by Cheri Pies, Spinsters Ink, 1988. Based on the author's very popular and ground-breaking workshop series for women considering becoming mamas, this is still the quintessential text to help you decide if you really want children in your life.

Lesbian and Gay Parenting Handbook: Creating and Raising Our Families by April Martin, Harper Perennial, 1993. A good primer on some of the issues facing gay and lesbian families. More issue-oriented, with little hard factual info on pregnancy or conception.

The Lesbian Parenting Book: A Guide to Creating Families and Raising Children by D. Merilee Clunis and G. Dorsey Green, Seal Press, 1995.

Lesbians Raising Sons edited by Jess Wells, Alyson Publications, 1997. With so many lesbians having sons, this anthology tries to answer the question of how our parenting of boys is different, and how our sons may be, too.

Women in Love: Portraits of Lesbian Mothers and their Families by Barbara Seyda with Diana Herrera, Bulfinch Press, 1998. Technically a coffee-table photo book, this striking collection of essays and images contains much wisdom on the beauty of lesbian families.

Waiting in the Wings: Portrait of a Queer Motherhood by Cherrie Moraga, Firebrand Books, 1997. A moving memoir about the premature birth of her son Rafael and their early life together.

Legal Issues for Lesbian Mamas

A Legal Guide for Lesbian and Gay Couples, 9th edition by Hayden Curry, Denis Clifford, and Robin Leonard, Nolo Press, 1996.

Lesbians Choosing Motherhood: Legal Implications of Alternative Insemination and Reproductive Technologies, 3rd edition, edited by Kate Kendell, National Center for Lesbian Rights, 1996. Available direct from NCLR (415) 392-6257.

Mainstream Books Worth a Mention

There are hundreds of pregnancy books on the market, but most contain nary a sentence about lesbian motherhood. Still, pregnancy does transcend marital and sexual status, if you can weed through the references to fathers and husbands. These are what I consider the best books of the bunch for their overall high quality of information mixed with general sensitivity to "alternative" lifestyles.

Complete Book of Pregnancy and Childbirth by Sheila Kitzinger, Knopf, 1996. Thoughtful, woman-centered book by a leading childbirth writer/educator. Good photos and a ton of medical information on pregnancy.

Your Pregnancy Week by Week by Glade Curtis, Fisher Books, 1997. For detail queens like me who had to know what the baby was doing and how it was growing and developing every week.

Parenting Guide to Pregnancy and Childbirth by Paula Spencer, Ballantine, 1998. One of the best pregnancy books I came across. Much better than the *What to Expect* book. This became my pregnancy Bible, because it contains information on every conceivable topic on pregnancy. If you can afford only one mainstream pregnancy book, I'd pick this one.

The Girlfriends' Guide to Pregnancy: Or Everything Your Doctor Won't Tell You by Nicole Iovine, Pocket Books, 1995. No, not written by "our" kind of girlfriend, but this book was one of the funniest and most right-on pregnancy books I read. Not content to soften symptoms, Iovine lets you know you'll be suffering but advises that the best remedy is to laugh.

What to Expect When You're Expecting by Arlene Eisenberg, Heidi E. Murkoff, and Sandee E. Hathaway, Workman Publishing, 1996. This phenomenally popular book was not my favorite, but you'll probably read it, since everyone else seems to! Good month-by-month information on your baby's in utero development.

Hip Mama Survival Guide: Advice from the Trenches on Pregnancy, Childbirth, Cool Names, Clueless Doctors, Potty Training and Toddler Avengers by Ariel Gore, Hyperion, 1998. Gore's alternative viewpoint is a welcome relief from the staunchiness and middle-class married perspective of most pregnancy books. Lots of info especially geared toward lower-income women. It's the kind of pregnancy book that's enjoyable reading even if you're not pregnant.

Natural Care

Wise Woman's Herbal for the Childbearing Year by Susun S. Weed, Ash Tree, 1985. How to use herbs during pregnancy to prevent miscarriage, curtail mood swings, control high blood pressure, and more. Also covers herbs for fertility and herbal remedies for babies. A fantastic resource!

Pocket Guide to Midwifery Care by Aviva Jill Romm, Crossing Press, 1998. A first primer on midwifery care, explaining who they are, what they do, and so on.

Becoming a Mom

Wanting a Child edited by Jill Bialosky and Helen Schulman, Farrar Straus & Giroux, 1998. A wonderful collection that accurately sums up baby lust and the efforts we will go to have a child. Some gay and lesbian contributors.

Child of Mine: Writers Talk About the First Year of Motherhood edited by Christina Baker Kline, Delta, 1998.

Past Due: A Story of Disability, Pregnancy, and Birth by Anne Finger. Seal Press, 1990.

Single Moms

The problem with most books on single motherhood is that they generally assume the woman is straight, got dumped by a man, and will somehow struggle on. As lesbian single mamas, we don't fit this pattern in the slightest, yet there may be some relevant information concerning finances, netwoking, and so on.

Operating Instructions: A Journal of My Son's First Year by Anne Lamott, Fawcett Books, 1994. Only one of my favorite books of all time! The journal-like quality of this memoir provides an intimate look into the world of Lamott's pregnancy and first year with her baby boy.

Two of Us Make a World: The Single Mother's Guide to Pregnancy, Childbirth and the First Year by Prudence and Sherill Tippins, Henry Holt, 1996. The book is a quickie overview of single-parenting issues from a straight woman's perspective.

Hip Mama Survival Guide (see above)

Breast-feeding

Breastfeeding Your Baby by Sheila Kitzinger, Knopf, 1998. Great photos and down-to-earth advice

The Nursing Mother's Companion, 4th edition, by Kathleen Huggins, Harvard Common Press, 1999. This is the book I found most helpful—the most detailed and useful on all aspects of breast-feeding.

The Womanly Art of Breastfeeding by La Leche League International, Plume, 1997. The "official" La Leche book.

Multiples

Having Twins: A Parent's Guide to Pregnancy, Birth and Early Childhood by Elizabeth Noble, Houghton Mifflin, 1991. Pregnancy, labor, and birth options if you're expecting twins.

Mothering Multiples, 2nd edition, by Karen Gromada, La Leche League, 1985. Twins on the way? This book covers the basics of how to cope and thrive! Available through the La Leche League (800) LA-LECHE.

Baby's Born—Now What?

There are a ton of books available on baby care. I'd recommend starting with the very thoughtful *The Baby Book: Everything You Need to Know About Your Baby from Birth to Age Two* by William and Martha Sears, Little Brown, 1993. Its emphasis on "attachment parenting" and following your instincts when parenting makes for a reassuring read. It also has lots of medical advice, advice for baby's first two years, and a great chapter on breastfeeding. For a good laugh at some of the emotional changes you may be going through as a new mama, check out *The Girlfriends' Guide to Surviving the First Year of Motherhood* by Vicki Iovine, Perigree, 1997. As with some of the others I've mentioned, this isn't a gay guidebook, but it is so woman-oriented that most dykes should be able to relate.

MAGAZINES

Gay Parent
Gay Parent is published every two months online at www.gayparentmag.com, as well as in print. Print version is available free at bookstores, community centers, and other establishments across the U.S.A. or by subscription ($18 for one year, $30 for two years).
Angeline Acain, Publisher
P.O. Box 750852 Forest Hills, New York 11375-0852
(718) 793-6641
gayparentmag@banet.net
www.gayparentmag.com

Alternative Family Magazine
By and for gay, lesbian, bisexual, and transgender parents and their children. Published bimonthly. Subscription: $24 per year.
Kelly Taylor, Publisher
P.O. Box 7179
Van Nuys, CA 91409
(818) 909-0314
Fax (818) 909-3792
altfammag@aol.com
www.altfammag.com

WEB SITES

AOL Lesbian Parenting
To reach the AOL lesbian parenting board, go to keyword OnQ. You'll find the Lesbian Parenting folder inside the Lesbian Discussion folder.

Family Q
www.studio8prod.com/familyq/
Family Q is a web resource for families headed by gays and lesbians, providing information on building and maintaining families. Includes a list of sperm banks.

Fertilitext Directory of Sperm Banks
www.fertilitext.org/
Fertilitext is a fertility treatment resource sponsored by Stadtlanders Pharmacy.

Lesbian Moms Web Page
www.lesbian.org/moms/index.htm
Information compiled by members of the lesbian moms' e-mail discussion list (for moms and mom wanna-bes) on topics including donors, insemination, health and diet, insurance, legal concerns, and adoption. Features a list of lesbian-friendly sperm banks.

Our Baby/Sharon's Home Page
www.nyu.edu/pages/sls/baby/baby.html
Home page of list wrangler Sharon Silverstein (see GLjewishparents and Moms-at-home) with links to many pregnancy and parenting resources.

SUPPLIES

Speculums
Check women's health centers, local area midwives, or places like Planned Parenthood for speculums. Plastic reusable speculums can also be mail ordered from Awakenings Birth Services.

Awakenings Birth Services
PO Box 14282
San Francisco, CA 94114
$7.95 plus $4 shipping in the U.S., $6 shipping to Canada. Write to them for shipping rates outside North America. Please make checks (in U.S. dollars) to Deborah Simone.

Bravado Designs
705 Pape Avenue
Toronto Ontario Canada M4K 3S6
(800) 590-7802
Fax (416) 466-8666
Bravado@idirect.com
web.idirect.com/~bravado/
Maternity underwear and nursing bras.

Motherwear
(800) 950-2500
info@motherwear.com
www.motherwear.com
Clothes for nursing mothers.

LESBIAN-FRIENDLY SPERM BANKS, HEALTH CLINICS, AND, FERTILITY RESOURCES

California Cryobank
Los Angeles Office (main office)
1019 Gayley Avenue
Los Angeles, CA 90024
(800) 231-3373
www.cryobank.com
California Cryobank maintains branch offices (listed below); however, orders are taken at and shipped from their main office.

Cambridge Lab
955 Massachusetts Avenue
Cambridge, MA 02139
(617) 497-8646
Palo Alto Lab
700 Welch Road, Suite 103
Palo Alto, CA 94304
(650) 324-1900

St. Louis Lab
11131 S. Towne Square, Suite H
St. Louis, MO 63123
(314) 894-2223

Fairfax Cryobank, USA
3015 Williams Dr, Suite #110
Fairfax, Virginia 22031
(800) 338-8407 or (703) 698-3976
Fax (703) 698-3933
cryobank@givf.com
www.fairfaxcryobank.com

Fenway Community Health Center
7 Haviland Street
Boston, MA 02115
(617) 267-0900
www.fchc.org/
Comprehensive, community-based health care clinic. Provides alternative insemination and other family and parenting services for lesbians, gay men, and bisexuals.

Growing Generations LLC
403 S. Bedford Dr.
Beverly Hills, CA 90212
(310) 551-1103
(310) 551-1133
family@growinggenerations.com
www.growinggenerations.com
Growing Generations is the first and only gay-and-lesbian-owned surrogacy firm exclusively serving the gay community worldwide. Growing Generations matches prospective parents with a surrogate and or egg donor and manages all aspects of the surrogacy process. Does not provide adoption or insemination services.

Lyon-Martin Women's Health Services
1748 Market St, Ste 201
San Francisco, CA 94102
Clinic: (415) 565-7667
Provides comprehensive health care
for women by women with a focus on
lesbians, women of color, low-income
women, older women, and women
with disabilities. Conducts forums,
workshops, and support groups for lesbian, gay, and bisexual parents and
prospective parents.

Pacific Reproductive Services
444 De Haro Street, Suite 222
San Francisco, CA 94107
(415) 487-2288
(888) 469-5800
Fax (415) 863-4358
Email pacifrepro@aol.com
www.hellobaby.com

Rainbow Flag Health Services and
Sperm Bank
(510) 763 - SPERM
(510) 763 - 7737
leland@gayspermbank.com
www.gayspermbank.com
Rainbow Flag Health Services and
Sperm Bank is the only sperm bank
that tells the mother who the donor is
when the child is three months old
and the first sperm bank in America to
accept gay donors. Located in
Oakland, California.

ReproMed Limited
56 Aberfoyle Crescent, Suite 209
Etobicoke, Ontario M8X 2W4
(416) 233-1212
Fax (416) 233-9180
info@repromedltd.com
www.repromedltd.com
Canadian sperm bank providing both
anonymous and known donor
options, along with in vitro fertilization
and direct sperm injection. Ships
sperm only to physicians.

Sperm Bank of California
2115 Milvia Street
Berkeley, CA 94704
(510) 841 1858
www.thespermbankofca.org

Xytex Corporation
1100 Emmett Street
Augusta, GA 30904
(800) 277-3210
xytex@xytex.com
www.xytex.com

MIDWIVES AND DOULAS

Association of Labor Assistants and Childbirth Educators (ALACE)
P.O. Box 382724
Cambridge, MA 02238
(888) 22-ALACE
(617) 441-2500
ALACE refers women to doulas, labor assistants, and childbirth classes. Their philosophy promotes "woman-centered" childbirth, using midwife care as the standard for safe and normal childbirth.

Doulas of North America (DONA)
(206) 324-5440
www.dona.com
AskDONA@aol.com
Contact DONA for a referral to a doula in your area.

Maia Midwifery and Preconception Services
Berkeley, CA 94703-2205
(510) 869.5141
maiamid@aol.com
www.maiamidwifery.com
Lesbian midwives who work mainly within the lesbian community. Midwifery service based in the San Francisco Bay Area also runs insemination support groups and childbirth classes for lesbians.

Midwives of North America (MANA)
An organization of North American midwives and their advocates whose central mission is to promote midwifery as a quality health care option for North American families.
4805 Lawrenceville Highway, Suite 116-279
Lilburn, GA 30047
info@mana.org
www.mana.org
1-888-923-MANA (6262)

MANA-Canada
Box 26141 RPO Sherbrook
Winnipeg, Manitoba
Canada R3C 4K9

SUPPORTIVE ORGANIZATIONS

Alternative Family Project
afp@thecity.sfsu.edu
www.queer.org/afp
(415) 436-9000
Fax (415) 431-6404
A multiservice, nonprofit, community-based agency for families with lesbian, gay, bisexual, or transgender members. Provides counseling and referrals.

Children of Lesbians and Gays
Everywhere (COLAGE)
3543 18th Street #17
San Francisco, CA 94110
(415) 861-KIDS (5437)
Fax (415) 255-8345
colage@colage.org
www.colage.org
COLAGE is the support and advocacy organization for daughters and sons of lesbian, gay, bisexual, and transgender parents.

The Family Pride Coalition
P.O. Box 34337
San Diego, CA 92163
(619) 296-0199
program@familypride.org
www.familypride.org
Founded in 1979, The Family Pride Coalition supports and protects the families of gay, lesbian, bisexual, and transgendered parents through advocacy, education, and direct service.

International Cesarean Awareness
Network (ICAN)
1304 Kingsdale Avenue
Redondo Beach, CA 90278
(310) 542-6400
Fax (310)542-5368
www.childbirth.org/ICAN
ICANinfo@aol.com

Lavender Families Resource Network
P.O. Box 21567
Seattle, WA 98111
(206) 325- 2643 voice/TTD
The group formerly known as Lesbian Mothers' National Defense Fund has changed its name to Lavender Families Resource Network. This organization was formed twenty years ago by twelve mothers to support lesbian mothers fighting for custody of their children. The services have expanded over the years to include support beyond lesbian mothers to include gay fathers, lesbian grandmothers, bisexual mothers, and transsexual parents in their fight against discrimination in parenting.

Lesbian Mothers Support Society
P.O. Box 61, Station M
Calgary, Alberta, Canada T2P 2G9
(403) 265-6433
highs@cadvision.com
www.lesbian.org/lesbian-moms/index.htm
Lesbian Mothers Support Society is a Canadian nonprofit group that strives to provide peer support for lesbian parents and their children, as well as those lesbians considering parenthood.

Momazons
PO Box 82069
Columbus, OH 43202
(614) 267-0193
www.glbnet.com/business/oh/col/Mom
azons/Momazons1.html
A national organization and referral network by and for lesbians choosing to
have children. Publishes a newsletter.

Montreal Lesbian Mothers Association
(514) 846-1543 or (514) 277-7052.
monicole@citenet.net
Bilingual organization of lesbian
mamas, mama wanna-bes and their
children, providing support and social
activities along with medical and legal
information for lesbian parents.

National Center for Lesbian Rights
870 Market Street, Suite 570
San Francisco, CA 94102
(415) 392-6257
www.nclrights.org
info@nclrights.org

Our Family, The Gay and Lesbian
Family Group
P.O. Box 13505
Berkeley, CA 94712-4505
(510) 540-7774 or (415) 206-0545
information@ourfamily.org
www.ourfamily.org
Our Family, The Gay and Lesbian
Family Group is the largest family
social organization in northern
California. Each month Our Family
presents events throughout the Bay
Area for our more than 260 member
families. Our Family also presents
workshops on many issues of interest

to the family community. Our Family
encourages prospective parents to network and find support with their
members who have created family in
many ways. The Grandparents, Aunts
& Uncles Program seeks to foster
extended families throughout the
community. Members support and
network with each other through an
e-mail list, Web site, and bimonthly
newsletter.

Prospective Queer Parents
wild@sfo.com
www.geocities.com/WestHollywood/3
373
Prospective Queer Parents maintains a
Web site and Internet mailing list for
lesbian, gay, bisexual, transgender, and
other supportive people interested in
discussing issues related to alternative
parenting and child raising.

RESOLVE
1310 Broadway
Somerville, MA 02144
(617) 623-0744
resolveinc@aol.com
www.resolve.org/
RESOLVE provides timely, compas-
sionate support and information to
individuals who are experiencing
infertility, through advocacy and
public education.

E-MAIL LISTS

Gljewishparents
Gljewishparents is an e-mail list for
gay, lesbian, bi, and transgender
Jewish parents and mom and dad
wanna-bes. It is a place to discuss all
aspects of glbt Jewish parenting.
Contact Gljewishparents@shamash.org

LIL
LIL is a mailing list for lesbians, our
partners, and our loved ones who are
experiencing infertility. LIL provides a
safe place for the exchange of information and support to help us cope
with the range of feelings we may
experience while on the roller-coaster
ride of infertility. For information on
how to subscribe, send the message in
the text of the e-mail:
info lil
to majordomo@queernet.org.

Moms
For lesbian moms, co-moms, and
mommy wanna-bes. For information
on how to subscribe, send the message in the text of the e-mail:
info moms
to majordomo@queernet.org.

Moms-at-home
Moms-at-home is an e-mail list for
lesbian at-home mothers. This is a
place to discuss the unique challenges
and rewards of all aspects of life as a
"stay-at-home" mom, including but
not limited to parenting issues. The
focus of this list is full-time stay-at-

home lesbian moms, but you are
welcome to join if you work from
home, work part time, or are
considering staying home full time
with your child or children. Bisexual
women who are at home caring for
children in a parenting relationship
with another woman are also
welcome. To subscribe, send a
request to majordomo@queernet.org.
In the body of your message, write:
subscribe moms-at-home. For
information on how to subscribe to
the mailing list, send the message in
the text of the e-mail:
info moms-at-home
to majordomo@queernet.org.

PQP
An Internet mailing list for prospective
queer parents (lesbian, gay, bisexual,
transgender, and their supporters).
Provides a forum for the exchange of
information and a social gathering
space for queer people who are interested in child raising and parenting.
The PQP mailing list is loosely associated with an organization called
Prospective Queer Parents in the San
Francisco Bay Area. Also maintains a
Web site:
www.geocities.com/WestHollywood/3
373. For information on how to subscribe to the mailing list, send the
message in the text of the e-mail:
info pqp
to majordomo@queernet.org.

SEXUALITY RESOURCES

National STD Hotline: (800) 227-8922

National AIDS Hotline: (800) 342-2437

Safer Sex Page
www.safersex.org
Features information on safer sex for
lesbians.

San Francisco Sex Information
www.sfsi.org
(415) 989-SFSI
Provides free, anonymous, accurate,
nonjudgmental information about sex.
Hotline hours are Monday through
Friday, 3:00 P.M. to 9:00 P.M. Pacific
Time.

Appendix

SAMPLE DONOR-RECIPIENT AGREEMENT ON DONOR INSEMINATION

This agreement is made this _____
day of _____ by and between
_____, hereafter
DONOR, and _____,
hereafter RECIPIENT, who may also be
referred to herein as the "parties."

NOW, THEREFORE, in consideration of the
promises of each other, DONOR and
RECIPIENT agree as follows:

1. Each clause of this AGREEMENT is
   separate and divisible from the
   others and, should a court refuse
   to enforce one or more clauses of
   this AGREEMENT, the others are
   still valid and in full force.

2. DONOR has agreed to provide his
   semen to RECIPIENT for the purpose
   of artificial insemination. The
   parties have further agreed that
   DONOR's semen may be frozen at the
   time of donation and may be used by
   RECIPIENT at a subsequent time.

3. In exchange, RECIPIENT has agreed
   to pay the sum of $_____ dollars
   to DONOR each and every time he
   makes a semen donation.

4. Each party is a single person who
   has never married.

5. Each party acknowledges and agrees
   that, during the calendar year
   _____, RECIPIENT is attempting to
   become pregnant through artificial
   insemination, and that such
   inseminations will continue until
   conception occurs.

6. Each party acknowledges and agrees
   that DONOR is providing his semen
   for the purpose of said artificial
   inseminations, and does so with
   clear understanding that he will
   not demand, request, or compel any

An acknowledgement of payment of an agreed upon fee in exchange for the semen:

The marital status of each party:

A statement indicating the artificial insemination was the procedure used:

Statement's acknowledging the relinquishment of the donor's parental rights and responsibilities:

Sample Known Doner Agreement provided by the National Center for Lesbian Rights. Reprinted with permission.

guardianship, custody, or visitation rights with any child(ren) resulting from the artificial insemination procedure. Further, DONOR acknowledges that he fully understood that he would have no parental rights whatsoever with said child(ren).

7. Each party acknowledges and agrees that RECIPIENT, through this AGREEMENT, has relinquished any and all rights that she might otherwise have to hold DONOR legally, financially, or emotionally responsible for any child(ren) that results form the artificial insemination procedure.

The designation that the recipient has authority to name the child:

8. Each party acknowledges and agrees that the sole authority to name any child(ren) resulting form the artificial insemination procedure shall rest with RECIPIENT.

An acknowledgement that the donor waives any right to be named on the child's birth certificate:

9. Each party acknowledges and agrees that there shall be no father named on the birth certificate of any child(ren) born from the artificial insemination procedure.

A statement that the donor's rights to bring a paternity suit have been relinquished:

10. Each party acknowledges and agrees that the use of a licensed physician to receive the semen donations, as well as the execution of this AGREEMENT, were specifically chosen to avoid any finding that the DONOR is the legal father of the child(ren) pursuant to (name and section number of state statute if applicable). Consistent with that purpose, each party has executed this AGREEMENT with the purpose of clarifying her or his intent to release and relinquish any and all rights she or he may have to bring a suit to establish the paternity of any child(ren) conceived through the procedure of artificial insemination.

The designation that the recipient has sole authority to appoint a guardian or authorize an adoption:

11. Each party covenants and agrees that, in light of the expectations of each party as stated above, RECIPIENT shall have absolute authority and power to appoint a guardian for her child(ren), and that the RECIPIENT and such guardian may act with sole discretion as to all legal, financial, medical, and emotional needs of said child(ren), without any involvement with or demands of authority from DONOR.

A statement of how the parties will deal with the identity of the donor:

12. Each party covenants and agrees that neither of them will identify the DONOR as the parent of the child(ren), nor will either of them reveal the identity of the DONOR to any of their respective relatives or to any individual without the express written consent of the other party.

13. Each party acknowledges and agrees that the relinquishment of all rights, as stated above, is final and irrevocable. DONOR further understands that his waivers shall prohibit action on his part for custody, guardianship, or visitation in any future situation, including the event of RECIPIENT's disability or death.

A statement concerning the donor's future contact with the child:

14. Each party acknowledges and agrees that any future contact the DONOR may have with any child(ren) that result(s) from the artificial insemination procedure in no way alters the effect of this agreement. Any such contact will be at the discretion of the RECIPIENT and will be consistent with the intent of both parties to sever any and all parental rights and responsibilities of the DONOR.

An acknowledgement that the parties understand that the agreement presents legal questions that are unsettled:

15. Each party acknowledges and understands that there may be legal questions raised by the issues involved in this AGREEMENT which

have not been settled by statute or prior court decisions. Notwithstanding the knowledge that certain of the clauses stated herein may not be enforced by a court of law, the parties choose to enter into this agreement.

A statement that each party signed the agreement voluntarily and freely:

16. Each party acknowledges and agrees that she or he signed this AGREEMENT voluntarily and freely, of his or her own choice, without any duress of any kind whatsoever. It is further acknowledged that each party has been advised to secure the advice and consent of an attorney of her or his own choosing, and that each party understands the meaning and significance of each provision of the AGREEMENT.

17. Each party acknowledges and agrees that any changes made in the terms and conditions of this AGREEMENT shall be made in writing and signed by both parties.

18. This AGREEMENT contains the entire understanding of the parties. There are no promises, understandings, agreements or representations between the parties other than those expressly stated in this AGREEMENT.

IN WITNESS WHEREOF, the parties hereunto have executed this AGREEMENT, consisting of_____ typewritten pages, in the City of_____, County of _____, State of California, on the date and year first written above.

_____   _____
DONOR   RECIPIENT

Basal Body Temperature Chart

Days of Cycle	1	2	3	4	5	6	7	8	9	10	11	12	13	14	15	16	17	18	19	20	21	22	23	24	25	26	27	28	29	30	31	32	33	34	35	36	37	38	39	40	41	42
Date of Month																																										
Spin																																										
Surge																																										
Menstruation																																										

99.0°
.8
.6
.4
.2
98.0°
.8
.6
.4
.2
97.0°

Basal Body Temperature Chart from *The Ultimate Guide to Pregnancy for Lesbians* by Rachel Pepper

Index

A

A and D ointment, 145
abortion, 8
acne, 91, 127
acupuncture, 23, 95
adoption, x, 76
AFP blood test, 118, 119
age, as risk factor in pregnancy, 8,
    104
AIDS, x
alcohol, 6, 34, 94, 118
Alpha-fetoprotein see AFP
Alternative Family, 65
America Online, xi
American Academy of Pediatrics,
    148
amniocentesis, 104, 119
amniotic fluid, 138, 153-154
amniotic sac, 153-154
anal bacteria, 7, 133
anal sex, 133
anemia, 119
anovulatory, 68, 71
appetite, 89
arnica, 147
arousal, 23
attachment parenting, 180-181
Awakenings Birth Services, 100, 134

B

baby care, 167, 183-184
Baby Bee cream, 145
baby oil, 7
baby shower, 143-144
basal body thermometer, 24
*Beginning Life: The Marvelous Journey
    from Conception to Birth*, 18
belly check, 108, 120
birth, 120, 161-162; complications,
    164; plan, 120; positions, 161;
    premature, 141
birth certificate, 122, 147
birth defects, 104
birthing center, 122
bisexual, ix
blastocyst, 18
bleeding, abnormal, 75; gums, 111
bloating, 109
blood type, 34
blood pressure, 101, 119
blood volume, 85
bloody show, 153
blue cohosh, 94
bondage, 133
bonding, with baby, 166, 167-169
books, ix, 64-65; baby care, 145,
    183; lesbian; xi,

mainstream, x-xi, 78, 126; sex guides, 130, 135
"Born on Foreign Soil," 169
bottle-feeding, 177, 179
Bravado Designs, 178,
Braxton-Hicks contractions, 112, 152
breast engorgement, 171, 177
breast-feeding, 116, 120, 175-179; advantages for baby, 175; pain, 176; and partners, 178
breast pump, 178
breasts, sore, 30, 79, 127, 171
Bright, Susie, 129, 130
bunting bag, 115

C

caffeine, 6, 22, 95, 118
calcium, 93, 109
calendula cream, 111
cancer, ovarian, 71
carbohydrates, 93
cervical mucus, see mucus
cervix, dilation, 152, 157-159; position, 20, 29, 158; and surge, 29
Cesarean section, 142, 145
chest pains, 141
childbirth classes, 139-140
China, adoption in, 76
Chinese teas, 22
chlamydia, 7, 13, 34, 75
chloasma, 112
chromosomes, 19, 104
chronic villus sampling, see CVS
circumcision, 148
Clearplan Easy, 28
clitoris, 130
Clomid, 14, 60, 71-73
clomiphene citrate see Clomid
CMV, 13, 34
Cole, Joanna, 123
colostrum, 177
conception, 16-18
Conception Technologies, 28
condoms, 7, 23
Considering Parenthood, 14

constipation, 92, 118
contractions, 141, 154-155; after orgasm, 135-136, 150
coparenting, 12, 41, 98-99, 115, 123-124, 182-183
cord, cutting 120
Cousins, Lucy, 123
cramps, 75
"crescent moon" position, 161
Crisco, 7
cunnilingus, 134
Curve, xi
CVS, 102
cystic fibrosis, 101
cytomegalovirus, see CMV

D

dairy, 92-93
day care, 115
debt, 4-5
deciding to parent, ix, 1-2, 76-77
dehydration, and cervical mucus, 22
delivery, estimated date of, 84
dental care, 111
DES, 72, 141
desire see sex drive
diabetes, 8-9
diapers, 115-116, 145
diarrhea, 141
diethylstillbestrol See DES
dieting, 23
dildos, 132-133
disability, and parenting, 10; and pregnancy, 8-10
donors, anonymous, x, 57; gay, 32; health screening, 34, 42; heterosexual, 32; known, 32- 41, 43-44; legal concerns, 36-39, 57; selecting, 35, 47-48; unknown, 32
doppler, 80
douching, 23
doula, 115, 121-122, 171-172
Doulas of North America, 122
Down's syndrome, 8, 101, 104, 119
Dreft, 115
drinking water, 6, 88, 139